PROOF AND CONCEPTS IN RAPID DIAGNOSTIC TESTS AND TECHNOLOGIES

Edited by **Shailendra K. Saxena**

Proof and Concepts in Rapid Diagnostic Tests and Technologies
http://dx.doi.org/10.5772/61405
Edited by Shailendra K. Saxena

Contributors

Theam Soon Lim, Angela Chiew Wen Ch'Ng, Paulo António Rodrigues Pereira, Guodong Sui, Cristina Petrisor, Manuela Sfichi, Nadia Gherman, Mihaela Cocis, Natalia Hagau, Maria Gazouli, Anna Lyberopoulou, Efstathios Efstathopoulos, David Gaze, John Sandoval, Lisa Van Houwelingen, Shailendra K. Saxena

Published by InTech

Janeza Trdine 9, 51000 Rijeka, Croatia

Publishing Process Manager Edi Lipovic

Technical Editor SPi Global

Cover InTech Design team

First published September, 2016

Printed in Croatia

Additional hard copies can be obtained from orders@intechopen.com

Proof and Concepts in Rapid Diagnostic Tests and Technologies, Edited by Shailendra K. Saxena

p. cm.

Print ISBN 978-953-51-2580-8
Online ISBN 978-953-51-2581-5

For EU product safety concerns:
IN TECH d.o.o., Prolaz Marije Krucifikse Kozulić 3, 51000 Rijeka, Croatia,
info@intechopen.com or visit our website at intechopen.com.

Meet the editor

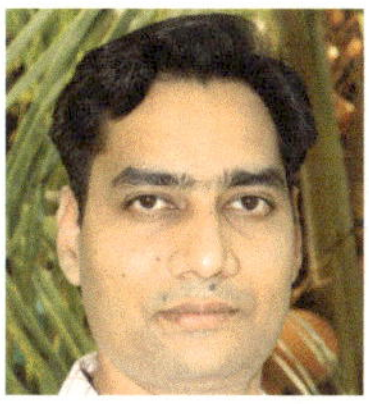

Prof. Shailendra K. Saxena is the Professor and Head of the Centre for Advance Research (CFAR), King George's Medical University (KGMU), Lucknow, India. His research interests are to understand the molecular mechanisms of host defense during human viral infections and to develop new predictive, preventive, and therapeutic strategies for them using JEV, HIV, and oncogenic viruses as a model, via stem cell and cell culture technologies. His research work has been published in various high-impact factor journals (*Science, PNAS, Nature Medicine*) with high citation. He has received many awards and honors in India and abroad including various Young Scientist Awards, BBSRC India Partnering Award and Fellows and is named as the Global Leader in Science by *The Scientist* magazine (USA) and International Opinion Leader/Expert involved in the vaccination for JE by IPIC (UK).

Contents

Preface

Diagnostic tests play a major role in the clinical care of patients. Whether caring for an individual patient with a disease/infection or responding to a worldwide pandemic, the rapid and accurate establishment of a cause is fundamental to quality care. Microscopy and other molecular-level diagnoses are time-tested standard tests for detection of diseases of humans and animals. On the other hand, it has firm limitations such as: requiring more time, human resources and the use of expensive equipments. A lot of research and development has focused on developing alternative methods for laboratory diagnosis and early detection of diseases. Antibodies and other serum components have been utilized successfully in a variety of diagnostic stands ranging from usual immunoassays to lateral flow assays, DNA-integrated assays, nanoparticles, microfluidics, and others.

Rapid diagnostic tests (RDTs) for diseases offer a new diagnostic alternative for health professionals and results from advances in chemistry, immunology, molecular biology, biochemistry, nucleic acid amplification, and engineering. The advent of recombinant antibody technology does not only allow for an earlier and more cost-effective answer for antibody generation but also offers diagnostic developers with the option to customize the antibodies.

Another approach for rapid diagnosis is by using flow cytometry, which helps in the detection of cell morphological changes such as granularity, size, etc. Detection of the expression of different cell surface and intracellular protein markers is also possible using flow cytometry during various abnormal conditions. RDTs are mainly based on the detection of antibodies, cytokines, and other serum components, which are specifically released during particular diseases.

Henceforth, keeping in mind all the issues, this book gives a comprehensive overview of the recent advancement and development of RDTs, which are quite new products and might be used as laboratory bench manual for the rapid diagnosis of the diseases.

The authors and editors of the book hope that this work might increase the interest in this field of research and that the readers will find it useful for their investigations, management, and clinical usage. Also I would like to thank Vice Chancellor, King George's Medical University (KGMU), Lucknow, colleagues, family, and parents who gave me a lot of encouragement and support during the work on this book.

Dr. Shailendra K. Saxena, PhD, DCAP, FAEB, FIVS, FBRS, FCMS
CSIR-Centre for Cellular and Molecular Biology,
India

Section 1

RDTs' in Diagnosis of Infectious Diseases

Chapter 1

Introductory Chapter: Serum Components as Rapid Diagnostic Biomakers During Flavivirus Infection

Shailendra K. Saxena and Sai V. Chitti

Additional information is available at the end of the chapter

http://dx.doi.org/10.5772/64784

1. Introduction

Infectious diseases are closely dependent on the nature and complexity of human behaviour, as they reflect who we are, what we do and how we interact with other people, animals and the environment. Worldwide, these diseases remain a leading source of human morbidity and mortality in all age groups [1]. Their emergence is thought to be driven largely by socio-economic, environmental and ecological factors [2]. According to Centre for Strategic and International studies, globally 16% of the deaths each year are from infectious diseases, this number not only causes huge burden but also produces immense challenge toward building better healthcare system. The past few years witnessed emergence and re-emergence of several microbial infections. A majority of them have been vector-borne infections (especially, the arthropod-borne) viral diseases, which constitute 90% of the re-emerging diseases [3]. Mosquito-borne *Flaviviruses* provide some of the most important examples of emerging and resurging diseases of global significance [4]. Virulent strains of these viruses are continually evolving and expanding their geographic range, thus rapid and sensitive screening assays are required to detect emerging viruses and monitor their prevalence and spread. Diagnostic tests play a major role in the clinical care of patients with infectious diseases, including detection of specific pathogens, discovery of new pathogens, determining appropriate therapy, monitoring response to therapy, assessing prognosis and disease surveillance. Whether caring for an individual patient with an infectious disease or responding to a worldwide pandemic, the rapid and the accurate establishment of a microbial cause is fundamental to quality care [5].

2. Flaviviruses

Flaviviruses are responsible for a number of important mosquito-borne diseases of man and animals globally. These are a highly diverse group of RNA viruses classified within the genus *Flavivirus,* family Flaviviridae [6]. *Flavivirus* includes >70 viruses, which are potent human pathogens [7]. These viruses are central etiologic agents of human disease, causing clinical disease ranging from fever to severe manifestations, such as encephalitis and hemorrhagic fever [8]. They are positive-stranded RNA viruses containing a genome of 10–11 kb. Genome is divided into three structural genes—the capsid (C), membrane (M) and envelope (E)—and seven non-structural (NS) genes—NS1, NS2A, NS2B, NS3, NS4A, NS4B and NS5 [9]. Growing cases of dengue virus (DV) and Japanese encephalitis virus (JEV) in Asia, recurrent outbreaks of yellow fever virus (YFV) in Africa and South America and the continuing spread of West Nile virus (WNV) all through the Americas show the geographical burden of *Flavivirus* diseases. These particular viral diseases are a significant burden on global economies and public health, including the recent Zika virus (ZIKV) and DV diseases, which caused emergency situation across the globe. Accurate diagnosis and differentiation of the infecting virus is important, especially in areas where many *Flaviviruses* are circulating [8].

3. Present flavivirus diagnostic test

Flavivirus diagnosis is often unclear the reason is that the laboratory diagnosis of these viral infections is based on isolation of the virus, detection of viral RNA using reverse transcription polymerase chain reaction (RT-PCR), plaque reduction neutralization test (PRNT), haemagglutination and haemagglutination inhibition assays (HI), antibody detection, immunofluorescence assays (IFA) and enzyme immunoassays (EIA), high-throughput, rapid microneutralisation assays, lateral flow assay (LFA), microsphere immunoassay (MIA), biosensors and microfluidic systems and autologous red blood cell agglutination assays [10]. Most of these assays results may not declare the specific *Flavivirus* infection, since most of them have cross-reactivity or the other issues.

4. Disadvantages of the available tests

The disadvantages of the present available tests include—For PRNT: labour intensive, require skilled personnel, a minimum of 5 days to perform and the handling of live virus, which requires a Biosafety level 3 (BSL-3) facilities. For HI: different pH buffers are required for each different antigen. A constant supply of fresh avian red blood cells is also necessary and there is a high level of cross-reactivity among the *Flaviviruses* [11]. For IFA: requirement for a fluorescent microscope to evaluate the results and cross-reactivity. For enzyme-linked immunosorbent assay (ELISA): unable to differentiate infections caused by different subtypes of particular *Flavivirus*. Accurate diagnosis and differentiation of the infecting virus is important, especially in areas where many *Flaviviruses* are circulating. For LFA: sample number should be small. For MIA: requires specialized equipment [12].

5. Need for rapid diagnosis

One of the major challenges during any outbreak is early diagnosis of infection, which is difficult because the early symptoms are non-specific toward particular infection and often are seen in patients with more common diseases [13]. During outbreaks, rapid detection of pathogens in individual cases is crucial in achieving the best clinical management, public health surveillance and control outcomes. With the addition of fields such as chemistry, immunology, molecular biology, biochemistry, nucleic acid amplification and engineering, it is now possible to determine the specific aetiology of a patient's infectious disease in the hospital, clinic, office, remote village or even a patient's home. With automation and highly multiplexed assays, individual pathogens can be readily identified in a wide variety of specimen types, including blood, urine, tissue, mucosal swabs, cerebrospinal fluid, respiratory secretions and stool samples. But one of the major limitations of all present available gold standard techniques is that they require time, which is not possible in case of deadly infectious diseases [5]. Therefore, rapid, accurate and accessible detection of infections have to be done. This has an important role in addressing not only mortality but also the spread of the disease into the newer areas. Rapid diagnostic tests (RDTs) offer the potential to provide accurate diagnosis to all at risk populations those unable to access services such as microscopic and other observation of the specimen. RDTs offer a useful alternative to microscopy.

5.1. Advantages of RDTs

- Personal exposure to patient sample is less.
- Maintaining a specialized laboratory with adequately skilled scientists, technicians and supportive personnel is not required.
- Very less use of high costly instruments and facilities.
- Resources and reagents requirement is limited.
- Discarding of the RDTs equipment is easy.

5.2. Limitations of RDTs

- Environmental conditions such as temperature and humidity can affect the performance of RDTs.
- Packaging, transport and storage are important for proper working of RDTs.

5.3. The ideal RDTs

The properties of RDTs kits play an enormous role in determining their utility in the diagnosis of infectious diseases. The prerequisites of the ideal RDTs include the following:

- Single step processing of the sample.
- Rapid and accurate results.
- RDTs should be cost-effective and sustainable in the long term.
- They have to replace with standard identification test.
- High sensitivity and specificity.
- Reproducible results.
- Purity and volume of assay sample.

6. Serum components as rapid diagnostic markers during flavivirus infections

The short vireamic period in infected hosts means that serological assays are often the diagnostic method of choice. Serum consists of substances that are produced mainly by the body in response to stress, diseases, pathogens, etc. In case of infectious diseases, a serological blood test is performed to detect and measure the levels of antibodies or other serum substances as a result of exposure to a particular microorganism [14]. Studies on serum proteome, cytokines and inflammatory markers during specific *Flavivirus* infection may give us clue for the development of rapid diagnosis. During *Flavivirus* infections since most of the cases are

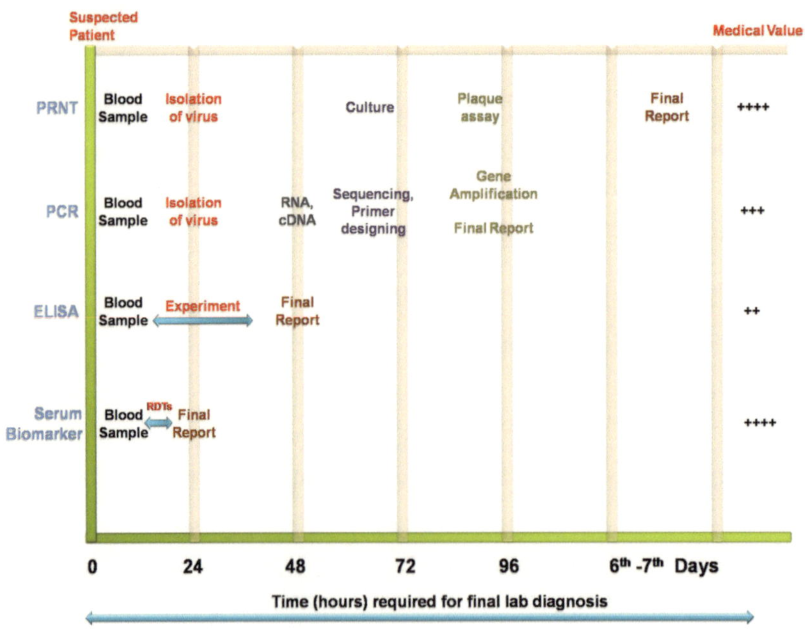

Figure 1. The time taken by the various diagnostic techniques for *Flavivirus* detection and their medical value. Compared to all other available techniques rapid diagnosis using serum offers the best approach to detect the specific *Flavivirus* infection.

asymptomatic during the early phase of the exposure, if the physician has to relay on techniques like PRNT, which is a time consuming, then patient may die, as few patients have short incubation period (**Figure 1**). Serum biomarker analysis for the particular infection and immediate treatment can help the patient to recover soon. The present most precise method for detecting *Flavivirus* infection is PRNT. Even though this method has great insight into this particular virus biology and pathogenesis, it has quite a few boundaries as discussed above. The main weakness that limits the clinical relevance of serological methods (if one is looking for IgG/IgM) is the broad antigenic cross-reactivity that exists between all *Flaviviruses*. The quite specific viral envelope (E) protein neutralizing antibody response may contribute to the false positive results since the amino acid sequences are more conserved. Hence looking for serum biomarkers (other than IgM, IgG) for particular infection can help in rapid diagnostics, least expensive and easy to perform. Here we list out few biomarkers (**Figure 2**) that are available till date for the detection of the *Flavivirus* infections.

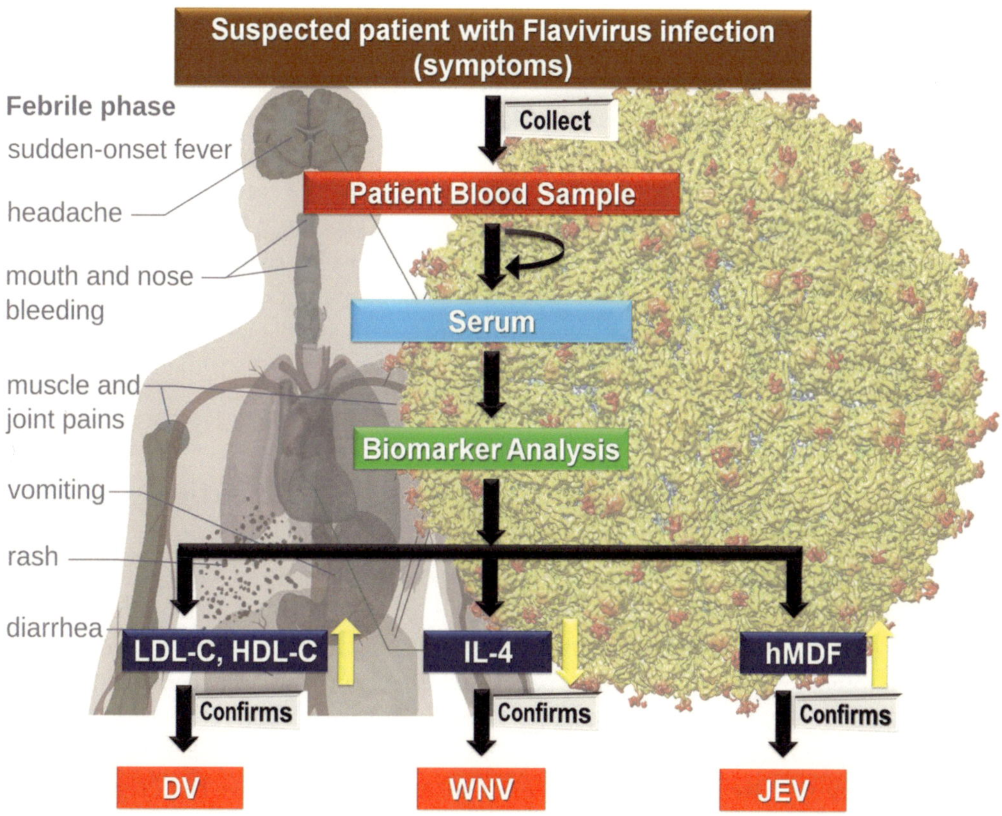

Figure 2. The rapid diagnosis procedure: When an individual with suspected *Flavivirus* infection approaches clinician. The clinician has to go for specific diagnosis based on the symptoms and travel history of the patient. Here are the precise serum biomarkers that are upregulated/downregulated during definite infection.

7. Cholesterol as prognostic biomarker during DV infection

Dengue is a systemic viral infection transmitted between humans by *Aedes* mosquitoes. DV is a *Flavivirus* of global importance, with about four billion people across 128 countries at possibility of infection, and 96 million clinically apparent cases predictable annually [15–17]. The clinical presentation of acute dengue infection is non-specific. The laboratory confirmation of dengue infection relies on isolation of the virus in cell culture, the identification of viral nucleic acid or antigens or the detection of virus specific antibodies [18]. The recent report suggests that the total serum cholesterol, low density lipoprotein (LDL-C) and high density lipoprotein (HDL-C) levels can be used as biomarker during dengue infection since these levels were considerably lower in dengue-positive patients compared to dengue-negative patients. The LDL-C levels showed larger decrease and thus may contribute to the reduction in total cholesterol. Liver damage caused by DV infection may possibly contribute to the lower cholesterol levels. It was also observed that total LDL-C and HDL-C levels were lower in severe compared to mild dengue. In conclusion, lower total serum cholesterol and LDL-C levels at presentation were associated with subsequent development of dengue hemorrhagic fever. In addition, the study also indicates that cholesterol level at presentation may serve as a probable forecaster of severe dengue [19]. Cholesterol and other routine laboratory markers should be explored as a lower cost and more sustainable move toward the development of biomarker that can serve as prognostic marker for dengue viral infection. Another study reported that serum angiopoietin-2 and soluble vascular endothelial growth factor receptor-2 (VEGFR-2) showed a strong correlation with the occurrence of plasma leakage in DV infected patients. It was also suggested they could serve as substitute markers for plasma leakage in patients with acute DV infection [20]. More work need to be done on these markers to confirm that these can be used in rapid diagnosis of dengue infection. There is an urgent need for the development of diagnostic and prognostic tools to identify dengue cases and to provide appropriate supportive care.

8. Serum cytokine profile as biomarker during WNV infection

WNV is a neurotropic human pathogen that is the causative agent of West Nile fever and encephalitis. From 1999 to 2012, 37,088 cases were reported to the US-Centers for Diseases Control, including 1549 fatalities [21]. About one in five people who are infected will develop a fever with other symptoms. Patients typically develop symptoms between 3 and 14 days after they are bitten by the infected mosquito. Centers for Disease Control and Prevention as of September 15, 2015, a total of 46 states in USA have reported WNV infections in people, birds or mosquitoes. Overall, 708 cases of WNV disease in people have been reported. The cumulative incidence of WNV infection may include as many as three million people [22]. The study on serum cytokines found that subjects with a history of severe infection had significantly lower levels of the serum IL-4, whereas asymptomatic subjects had elevated baseline levels of the IL-4 [23]. The study on serum protein profile of healthy and virus infected individual may give us clue on biomarker discovery and to develop serum based diagnosis of the WNV infection.

9. Diagnosis of St. Louis encephalitis virus

St. Louis encephalitis virus (SLEV) was the leading cause of epidemic *Flaviviral* encephalitis in the United States prior to the introduction of WNV in late 1999 [24, 25]. Preliminary diagnosis is often based on the patient's clinical features, places and dates of travel, activities and epidemiologic history of the location where infection occurred. Majority of SLEV infections remain undiagnosed since the symptoms are like normal flu illness [26]. A standardized IgM antibody-capture enzyme-linked immunosorbent assay protocol is the only available diagnosis for SLEV infection [27]. This assay serves as a priceless tool for the presumptive diagnosis of acute SLEV infections and facilitates the processing of many serum samples. But, the major drawback of this assay is that during the antigen preparation from virus-infected suckling mouse brain the personnel may expose to infectious agents and hazardous chemicals. In addition, the procedure for this antigen preparation is time consuming, costly and tedious [28]. Research need to emphasize on development of rapid diagnosis kit that aids on identification of SLEV at much earlier stage.

10. Serum protein profile as biomarker during JEV infection

According to WHO, global health observatory data repository, there were 4707 reported number of JEV infection cases in 2014 [29]. Japanese encephalitis (JE) is an acute viral zoonotic infection of the central nervous system (CNS), which produces meningomyeloencephalitis. It poses a serious public health problem with an increasing frequency of epidemics and outbreaks in many parts of the Indian subcontinent and Southeast Asian countries [30, 31]. The preliminary diagnosis of JEV is often based on the patient's clinical features, places and dates of travel. The present laboratory diagnosis of JE is generally accomplished by testing of serum or cerebrospinal fluid (CSF) to detect virus-specific IgM antibodies. JEV IgM antibodies are usually detectable 3–8 days after onset of illness and persist for 30–90 days. But the main weakness that limits the clinical relevance of these methods is the broad antigenic cross-reactivity that exists between all *Flaviviruses* and this may contribute to the false positive results. Serum protein profiles other than antibodies work as potential biomarkers for knowing disease status. The analysis of serum proteins of patients and healthy individual by surface-enhanced laser desorption/ionization–time of flight–mass spectrometry (SELDI-TOF-MS) in combination with the ProteoMiner technology that accurately displays low-abundance proteins responsible for virus infection could help physicians for rapid diagnosis of JEV infection [32]. One of the serum factors that could serve as potential biomarker is human macrophage-derived factor (hMDF) that specifically secreted during JEV infection. The levels of hMDF in blood will rise to its highest level by second week of infection [33, 34]. Hence, the detection of hMDF in blood could be a useful prognostic marker of the JEV infection.

11. Conclusion

The burden of *Flaviviral* infection is expected to continue to increase in the future due to climate change, globalization, travel, trade, urbanization, socioeconomics, viral evolution and other factors. The short incubation time for most of the *Flaviviruses* infections and no specific diagnosis make these an important public health problem globally. RDTs methods may be implemented as adjuncts to the epidemiologic investigation of *Flavivirus* disease outbreaks. As sensitivities, specificities, positive predictive value and negative predictive value of RDTs continue to improve and become more widely appreciated through production of less expensive and more user-friendly platforms, it will become necessary to formulate responsible guidelines for the appropriate and optimal use in clinical practice in clarifying infectious disease diagnoses and improving patient outcomes. There is a critical call for discovery of serum biomarkers that are specifically present or up-regulated during particular *Flavivirus* infection. Recently, there were many reports on micro-RNA (miRNA), which gets upregulated or downregulated during these particular infections but relaying on miRNA may not be the right practice since they are regulated by several factors and it involves molecular biology work and equipment. The advantage of serum analysis is that, it is least expensive, easy to perform and biosafety practices are not required. Growing cases of *Flavivirus* infections globally says that there is a critical need for the development of diagnostic and prognostic tools to identify specific cases and to provide appropriate supportive care and with anticipation that one day there will be a specific diagnosis and therapeutics for all *Flavivirus* infection.

Acknowledgements

The authors are grateful to the Vice Chancellor, King George's Medical University (KGMU), Lucknow and Director, Centre for Cellular and Molecular Biology and Council of Scientific and Industrial Research (CSIR-CCMB), India for the encouragement and support for this work. SK Saxena is also supported by US National Institute of Health Grants: R37DA025576 and R01MH085259.

Author details

Shailendra K. Saxena[1,2*] and Sai V. Chitti[2]

*Address all correspondence to: shailen@ccmb.res.in and shailen1@gmail.com

1 Centre for Advance Research (CFAR), King George's Medical University (KGMU), Lucknow, Uttar Pradesh, India

2 CSIR-Centre for Cellular and Molecular Biology (CCMB), Hyderabad, Telangana, India

References

[1] Johnson PT, de Roode JC, Fenton A. Why infectious disease research needs community ecology. Science. 2015;349(6252):1259504. DOI:10.1126/science.1259504

[2] Jones KE, Patel NG, Levy MA, Storeygard A, Balk D, Gittleman JL, Daszak P. Global trends in emerging infectious diseases. Nature. 2008;451(7181):990–993. DOI: 10.1038/nature06536.

[3] Pattnaik P, Srivastava A, Abhyankar A, Dash PK, Parida MM, Lakshmana Rao PV. Fusogenic peptide as diagnostic marker for detection of flaviviruses. J Postgrad Med. 2006;52(3):174–178.

[4] Mackenzie JS, Gubler DJ, Petersen LR. Emerging flaviviruses: the spread and resurgence of Japanese encephalitis, West Nile and dengue viruses. Nat Med. 2004;10:98–109.

[5] Caliendo AM, Gilbert DN, Ginocchio CC, Hanson KE, May L, Quinn TC, Tenover FC, Alland D, Blaschke AJ, Bonomo RA, Carroll KC, Ferraro MJ, Hirschhorn LR, Joseph WP, Karchmer T, MacIntyre AT, Reller LB, Jackson AF; Infectious Diseases Society of America (IDSA). Better tests, better care: improved diagnostics for infectious diseases. Clin Infect Dis. 2013;57:39–170. DOI: 10.1093/cid/cit578.

[6] Grant-Klein RJ, Baldwin CD, Turell MJ, Rossi CA, Li F, Lovari R, Crowder CD,Matthews HE, Rounds MA, Eshoo MW, Blyn LB, Ecker DJ, Sampath R, Whitehouse CA.Rapid identification of vector-borne flaviviruses by mass spectrometry. Mol Cell Probes. 2010;24(4):219–228. DOI: 10.1016/j.mcp.2010.04.003.

[7] Saxena SK, Tiwari S, Swamy ML. An insight into flaviviral budding: a need to know more. Future Microbiol. 2014;9(2):125–128. DOI: 10.2217/fmb.13.151.

[8] Koraka P, Zeller H, Niedrig M, Osterhaus AD, Groen J. Reactivity of serum samples from patients with a flavivirus infection measured by immunofluorescence assay and ELISA. Microbes Infect. 2002;4(12):1209–1215.

[9] Tiwari S, Chitti SVP, Mathur A, Saxena SK. Japanese encephalitis virus: an emerging pathogen. Am J Virol. 2012;1:1–8.

[10] Sekaran SD, Artsob H. Molecular diagnostics for the detection of human flavivirus infections. Expert Opin Med Diagn. 2007;1(4):521–530. DOI: 10.1517/17530059.1.4.521.

[11] Endy TP, Nisalak A. Japanese encephalitis virus: ecology and epidemiology.Curr Top Microbiol Immunol. 2002;267:11–48.

[12] Hobson-Peters J. Approaches for the development of rapid serological assays for surveillance and diagnosis of infections caused by zoonotic flaviviruses of the Japanese encephalitis virus serocomplex. J Biomed Biotechnol. 2012;2012:379738, DOI: 10.1155/2012/379738.

[13] Koenig KL, Majestic C, Burns MJ. Ebola virus disease: essential public health principles for clinicians. West J Emerg Med. 2014;15(7):728–731. DOI:10.5811/westjem.2014.9.24011.

[14] Koene MG, Mulder HA, Stockhofe-Zurwieden N, Kruijt L, Smits MA. Serum protein profiles as potential biomarkers for infectious disease status in pigs. BMC Vet Res. 2012;8:32. DOI: 10.1186/1746-6148-8-32.

[15] Brady OJ, Gething PW, Bhatt S, Messina JP, Brownstein JS, Hoen AG, Moyes CL, Farlow AW, Scott TW, Hay SI. Refining the global spatial limits of dengue virus transmission by evidence-based consensus. PLoS Negl Trop Dis. 2012;6(8). DOI: 10.1371/journal.pntd.0001760.

[16] Simmons CP, Farrar JJ, Nguyen VV, Wills B. Dengue. N Engl J Med. 2012;366(15):1423–1432. DOI: 10.1056/NEJMra1110265.

[17] Bhatt S, Gething PW, Brady OJ, Messina JP, Farlow AW, Moyes CL, Drake JM,Brownstein JS, Hoen AG, Sankoh O, Myers MF, George DB, Jaenisch T, Wint GR,Simmons CP, Scott TW, Farrar JJ, Hay SI. The global distribution and burden of dengue. Nature. 2013;496(7446):504–507. DOI: 10.1038/nature12060.

[18] Peeling RW, Artsob H, Pelegrino JL, Buchy P, Cardosa MJ, Devi S, Enria DA,Farrar J, Gubler DJ, Guzman MG, Halstead SB, Hunsperger E, Kliks S, Margolis HS, Nathanson CM, Nguyen VC, Rizzo N, Vázquez S, Yoksan S. Evaluation of diagnostic tests: dengue. Nat Rev Microbiol. 2010;8:30–38.

[19] Biswas HH, Gordon A, Nuñez A, Perez MA, Balmaseda A, Harris E. Lower low-density lipoprotein cholesterol levels are associated with severe dengue outcome. PLoS Negl Trop Dis. 2015;9(9):e0003904. DOI: 10.1371/journal.

[20] van de Weg CA, Pannuti CS, van den Ham HJ, de Araújo ES, Boas LS, Felix AC,Carvalho KI, Levi JE, Romano CM, Centrone CC, Rodrigues CL, Luna E, van Gorp EC, Osterhaus AD, Kallas EG, Martina BE. Serum angiopoietin-2 and soluble VEGF receptor 2 are surrogate markers for plasma leakage in patients with acute dengue virus infection. J Clin Virol. 2014;60(4):328–335. DOI: 10.1016/j.jcv.2014.05.001

[21] Petersen LR, Carson PJ, Biggerstaff BJ, Custer B, Borchardt SM, Busch MP. Estimated cumulative incidence of West Nile virus infection in US adults,1999–2010. Epidemiol Infect. 2013;141(3):591–595. DOI: 10.1017/S0950268812001070

[22] Centers for Disease Control and Prevention. West Nile Virus (WNV) Fact Sheet. 2015. http://www.cdc.gov/westnile/resources/pdfs/wnvFactsheet_508.pdf

[23] Qian F, Thakar J, Yuan X, Nolan M, Murray KO, Lee WT, Wong SJ, Meng H, Fikrig E, Kleinstein SH, Montgomery RR. Immune markers associated with host susceptibility to infection with West Nile virus. Viral Immunol. 2014;27(2):39–47. DOI: 10.1089/vim.2013.0074

[24] Anderson JF, Andreadis TG, Vossbrinck CR, Tirrell S, Wakem EM, French RA,Garmendia AE, Van Kruiningen HJ. Isolation of West Nile virus from mosquitoes,crows, and a Cooper's hawk in Connecticut. Science. 1999;286(5448):2331–2333.

[25] Briese T, Jia XY, Huang C, Grady LJ, Lipkin WI. Identification of a Kunjin/West Nile-like flavivirus in brains of patients with New York encephalitis. Lancet. 1999;354(9186): 1261–1262.

[26] Terzian AC, Mondini A, Bronzoni RV, Drumond BP, Ferro BP, Cabrera EM, Figueiredo LT, Chiaravalloti-Neto F, Nogueira ML. Detection of Saint Louis encephalitis virus in dengue-suspected cases during a dengue 3 outbreak. Vector Borne Zoonotic Dis. 2011;11(3):291–300. DOI: 10.1089/vbz.2009.0200

[27] Martin DA, Muth DA, Brown T, Johnson AJ, Karabatsos N, Roehrig JT. Standardization of immunoglobulin M capture enzyme-linked immunosorbent assays for routine diagnosis of arboviral infections. J Clin Microbiol. 2000;38(5):1823–1826.

[28] Purdy DE, Noga AJ, Chang GJ. Noninfectious recombinant antigen for detection of St. Louis encephalitis virus-specific antibodies in serum by enzyme-linked immunosorbent assay. J Clin Microbiol. 2004;42(10):4709–4717.

[29] World Health Organisation. Global Health Observatory data repository. 2015. http://apps.who.int/gho/data/view.main.1520?lang=en

[30] Saxena SK, Mishra N, Saxena R, Singh M, Mathur A. Trend of Japanese encephalitis in North India: evidence from thirty-eight acute encephalitis cases and appraisal of niceties. J Infect Dev Ctries. 2009;3(7):517–530.

[31] Noronha N, Swamy MLA, Saxena SK. Japanese encephalitis: a major public-health debacle. Future Virol. 2014;9(10):883–886 , DOI 10.2217/fvl.14.75.

[32] Kant Upadhyay R. Biomarkers in Japanese encephalitis: a review. Biomed Res Int. 2013;2013: 591290, DOI: 10.1155/2013/591290.

[33] Srivastava S, Khanna N, Saxena SK, Singh A, Mathur A, Dhole TN. Degradation of Japanese encephalitis virus by neutrophils. Int J Exp Pathol. 1999;80(1):17–24.

[34] Singh A, Kulshreshtha R, Mathur A. Detection of a neutrophil chemotactic factor in Japanese encephalitis patients. J Pharm Sci Innov. 2012;1(6):23–26.

Section 2

RDTs' in Diagnosis of Cardiovascular Diseases

Chapter 2

Rapid Cardiovascular Diagnostics

David C. Gaze

Additional information is available at the end of the chapter

http://dx.doi.org/10.5772/63910

Abstract

Rapid cardiovascular diagnostics have played an integral role in the development of the clinical utility of cardiac biomarkers. Rapid qualitative and quantitative tests are used as an alternative to clinical chemistry laboratories, where urgent testing for cardiac biomarkers has been unavailable. Biomarkers are clinically available for diagnosis and prognosis across the heart disease continuum. Early risk markers of plaque formation and destabilisation are non-urgent and can be performed routinely as part of the pathology laboratory repertoire. Rapid diagnostic tests are best suited for markers of ischaemia, necrosis and heart failure, where patients often present acutely to emergency medical services. This chapter reviews the evolution of rapid cardiovascular diagnostics both in the pre-hospital and emergency department setting, compared to the utility of centralised laboratory testing. Further, limitations to their use and improvements by novel technology are discussed.

Keywords: cardiovascular disease, cardiac markers, cardiac troponin, centralised laboratory testing, ischemia, natriuretic peptides, rapid tests

1. Introduction

Cardiovascular disease (CVD) is the leading cause of death in the Western World with rates for coronary heart disease and stroke-related mortality exceeding that of any cancer. Patients who present to the emergency department (ED) with chest pain are often a complex clinical challenge. Classical electrocardiographic (ECG) changes of an acute cardiac episode occur in only 5–15% of ED presentations. Blood-borne biomarkers offer an alternative diagnostic mode and have been part of the clinical testing repertoire since the 1950s.

Cardiac biomarker testing can be performed in a spectrum of clinical settings. Normally, this occurs in a centralised laboratory, where blood is drawn from the patient and transported either by hand or pneumatic delivery chutes (**Figure 1**). The samples are processed in the laboratory along with other patient samples received from inpatients, outpatient clinics or from primary care. The combination of samples and the utility of multidisciplinary pathology laboratories can result in a time delay from drawing the sample to obtaining the results in the clinical setting (**Figure 2**).

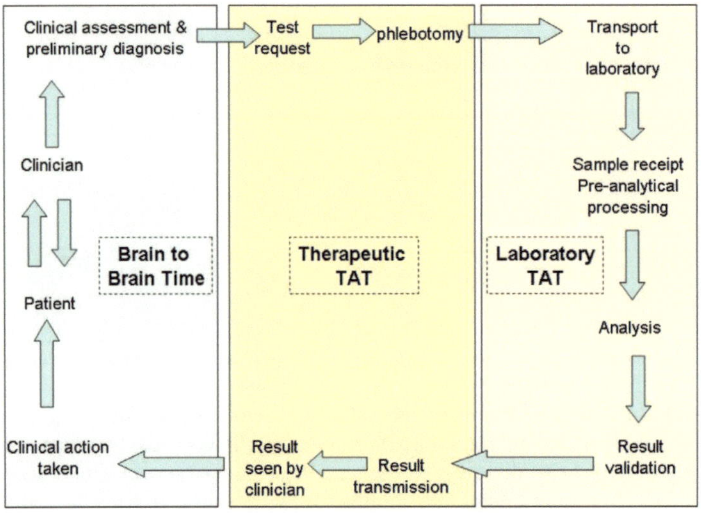

Figure 1. Cycle of delivery of diagnostic testing results. TAT, turnaround time.

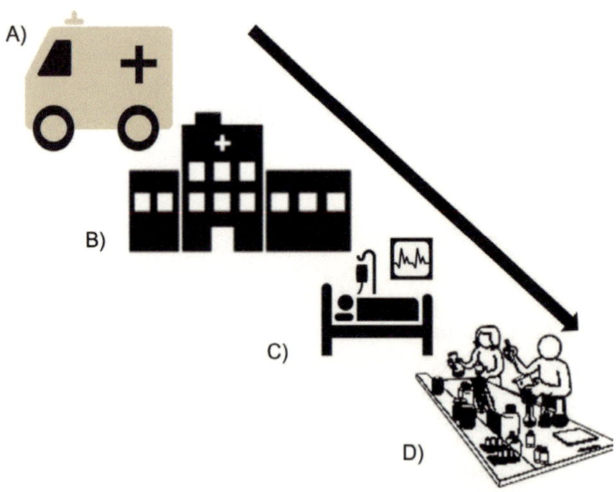

Figure 2. Cardiac biomarker testing. Testing can be performed in a number of settings including (A) pre-hospital by paramedical and ambulance personnel, (B) in a hot or STAT laboratory in the Emergency Department, (C) in the point of care setting such as the ED cubicle, patient bay or bedside or as is most conventional and (D) in a centralised clinical chemistry laboratory.

http://dx.doi.org/10.5772/63910

1.1. Point of care testing

The alternative to centralised laboratory testing is point of care testing (POCT). This has been known by many names and acronyms including near-patient testing; bedside testing; physicians' office testing; extra-laboratory, satellite 'hot lab'; decentralised laboratory; ancillary laboratory; or alternate site testing. Essentially, the aim of POCT analysis is to perform diagnostic laboratory tests with a shorter turnaround time (STAT) than that obtained by the central laboratory.

POCT is the ***immediate*** provision of a test ***at the point of healthcare delivery*** when the result will be used to make a decision and to take appropriate action, which leads to an improved health outcome [1]. POCT is not a novel concept, mentioned early in the foundation of medicine by Hippocrates (c. 460-370BC) and Galen (129-c.200AD). It was also described in the seventh century by the Byzantine physician Theophilus Protospatharius, a forerunner of modern Urology. Theophilus used uroscopy, the practice of visually examining patients urine with a urine flask and determining disease using the urine wheel; a colour chart of 20 urine flasks aligned in a circle and acts as a reference to link urine colour to particular diseases.

POCT can be useful for diagnosis (e.g. D-dimer or troponin in deep vein thrombosis and cardiac presentations), as a treatment guide or to monitor success of therapy (e.g. glucose/HbA1c in diabetes), in patient-related use (e.g. guidance and convenience of home INR and white cell count) and in physician-related factors (e.g. primary care natriuretic peptide testing to guide therapy in chronic heart failure). There are many advantages and disadvantages of using POCT over central laboratory services and these are given in **Table 1**.

Advantages	Disadvantages
Simpler sample collection (often finger prick)	Increased workload
Simpler pre-analytical handling	Increased error rate
Faster test results	Incompatibility if different laboratory methods used, e.g. clinical cut-off values
Reduces pathology access barriers	Increased cost
Increased patient satisfaction and user experience	Inadequate storage of results

Table 1. Advantages and disadvantages of point of care testing.

The most successful case in point for POCT is the use of glucose monitoring by finger prick testing. This has successfully revolutionised the management of diabetes both in the clinical scenario but more importantly in the patient's home. Other examples exist such as urine test strips for multiple analytes such as haemoglobin, reducing sugars, ketones, pH; human chorionic gonadotrophin (HCG) testing in home pregnancy testing kits; blood gas and electrolyte analysis; cholesterol testing in pharmacies, international normalised ratio (INR) for patients on warfarin anticoagulation therapy; rapid drugs of abuse screening in police custody or the ED; procalcitonin and c-reactive protein for rapid detection of sepsis; and human immunodeficiency virus in salivary samples.

The driver for adopting successful POCT is a balance between meeting realistic clinical need with the appropriate technology at a sensible cost. The overwhelming utility for POCT is the rapid delivery of results. This is appropriate for acute conditions, such as cardiac or respiratory events, ectopic pregnancy and sepsis. The other need is for diagnosis outside of standard clinical areas, such as monitoring in the patients home, testing in specialised walk-in centres (HIV testing) or in social care (drugs of abuse).

1.2. Analytical actuary and precision of point of care testing

Methods employed for POCT need to demonstrate adequate analytical performance with acceptable accuracy and precision in comparison to centralised laboratory methods. Obtaining results faster is of very limited value if the coefficient of variation (CV) for the analyte is excessively large (e.g. 25%) compared to a central laboratory method with a CV of 5% at the same concentration. It is generally accepted that the performance of POCT is limited compared to central laboratory testing due to constraints such as the technology employed, knowledge and training of users who are often non-laboratory trained and inadequate quality assurance monitoring.

Performance has been well documented for blood gas analysis [2–5], cholesterol determination on eight POCT systems [6] and for INR [7] as determined on the popular CoaguCheck XS device, which was highly comparable ($r = 0.91$) to a laboratory-based method.

1.3. Effect of point of care testing on turnaround time

There have been many studies investigating the effect of POCT usage on turnaround time (TAT). TAT for activated partial thromboplastin time in a centralised laboratory can take 45–60 min to complete yet 5–10 min by POCT [8, 9]. Blood gas analysis can be reduced from 25 min to approximately 13 min [10]. Collinson and colleagues [11] demonstrated improved TAT with cardiac marker testing by POCT compared to central laboratory testing. Typical laboratory and POCT TAT for common parameters are given in **Table 2**.

Analyte	Laboratory TAT (min)	POCT TAT (min)	ΔTAT (min)
Urinalysis	40	4	-36
βHCG (pregnancy)	78	5	-73
Glucose	10	6	-4
Cardiac markers	110	17	-93

Table 2. Commonly achieved turnaround times (TAT) for central laboratory or point of care testing (POCT).

http://dx.doi.org/10.5772/63910

1.4. Impact on patient care

Having an analytically sound and faster method of determining an analyte is all well and good; however, the final piece of the jigsaw is the translation into improvement of patient management and outcome over and above that of the central laboratory.

Parvin et al. [12] investigated the effect of routine use of POCT by non-laboratory personnel in the ED on length of stay. A handheld device was used to determine Na, K, Cl, glucose and urea. There was no relevant decrease in length of stay in the ED. In a UK study of 1728 patients, changes in patient management are made earlier for those who received POCT haematology testing (74 min earlier) and biochemical testing (21 min earlier) reducing the time to decision affecting patient management [13]. However, such changes did not affect clinical outcome or length of stay in the ED.

Specifically, for cardiac markers, on the basis of 263 admissions with chest pain, Collinson et al. [11] have demonstrated that patients who received POCT had a reduced length of stay, both in the coronary care unit and overall hospital stay compared to those who received conventional biomarker testing provided by the central laboratory. This final important step has played a pivotal role in the adoption (or lack of) of rapid cardiovascular diagnostics by POCT and is the focus of the remainder of this chapter.

2. Cardiovascular disease epidemiology

CVD is the leading cause of global death. World Heart Federation statistics demonstrate that 17.1 million deaths globally each year are due to CVD, with 82% occurring in the developing world. Such numbers are often difficult to comprehend. One in every five deaths in the USA is due to CVD. Thirty-five per cent of UK people <65 years old die prematurely due to CVD daily. Data prediction suggests that 23 million people will die annually from CVD by the year 2030.

2.1. Acute chest pain

The largest category of patients admitted to UK hospitals is due to chest pain [14]. Patients with chest pain are diagnostically challenging. The majority present with either stable ischaemic heart disease (IHD) or no IHD [15]. Such admissions are either clinically inappropriate or are of short duration, lasting hours or a few days maximum. However, 2–7% of patients with acute myocardial infarction (AMI) are inappropriately discharged from the ED [16, 17]. Improvements to diagnosis have been made utilising risk scoring systems [18], computerised decision support [19, 20] and automated ECG interpretation [21]. Although clinical assessment is paramount in the assessment of chest pain, cardiac biomarker measurements are now routinely used to aid diagnosis.

2.2. Cardiac biomarkers: a historical perspective

Since the early 1950s, the measurement of serum enzymes in the plasma following myocyte cell necrosis initially by activity then as mass concentration progressively became commonplace in the routine clinical laboratory. The utility of cardiac biomarkers in AMI was first introduced in 1954, with subsequent identification of biomarkers of infarction and ischaemia (**Figure 3**). Classical enzymatic cardiac biomarkers, such as aspartate transaminase (AST), lactate dehydrogenase (LDH) and creatine kinase (CK) and its MB isoform (CK-MB), or the muscle protein, myoglobin, were the front-line routine diagnostic tests for the larger part of 20 years. These, however, all demonstrated poor clinical utility, due to specificity. The majority of these enzymes and proteins had similar distribution and concentrations in both cardiac muscle cells and skeletal muscle. CK-MB proved superior of all the early markers and became the gold standard test for the diagnosis of AMI.

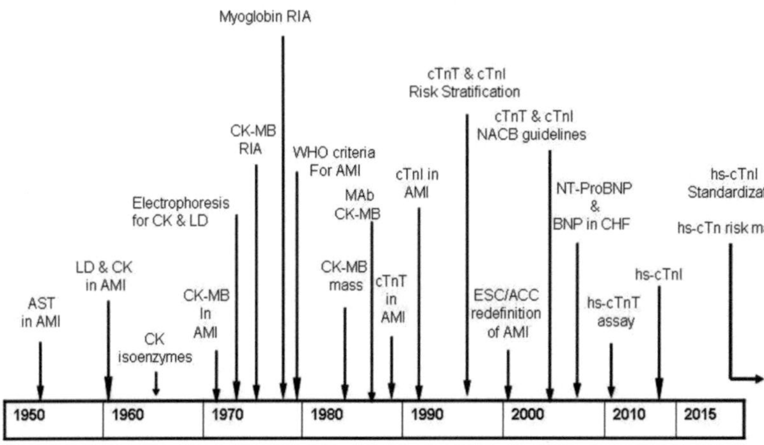

Figure 3. Historical chronology of biomarkers for the assessment of acute coronary syndrome. AMI, acute myocardial infarction; ACC, American College of Cardiology; AST, aspartate transaminase; BNP, B-type natriuretic peptide; CK, creatine kinase; CK-MB, creatine kinase-MB isoform; cTn, cardiac troponin; cTnI, cardiac troponin I; cTnT, cardiac troponin T; ESC, European Society of Cardiology; MAb, monoclonal antibody; NACB, National Academy of Clinical Biochemistry; NTproBNP, N-terminal pro-B-type natriuretic peptide; WHO, World Health Organisation. (Adapted with permission from Gaze and Collinson [22]).

Since the early 2000s, cardiac troponin T (cTnT) and I (cTnI) have become the universal gold standard test for the diagnosis of acute coronary syndrome (ACS) in those patients who present with chest pain and non-ST segment elevation on the ECG. ACS is a spectrum of disease ranging from unstable angina following an episode of cardiac ischemia to full thickness acute myocardial infarction (AMI) due to total occlusion of a coronary artery.

There have been numerous attempts to characterise the disease progression associated with CVD using different biomarkers targeting specific pathophysiological mechanisms. In patients who are asymptomatic, there are a number of biochemical tests that can be used to assess cardiovascular risk (**Table 3**). These are broadly categorised into those that assess plaque formation such as the lipid profile too assess vascular risk and metabolic markers associated

http://dx.doi.org/10.5772/63910

with obesity. As the pathological processes of atherosclerosis advances, markers are available to establish vulnerable culprit lesions in the coronary circuit. These markers of plaque destabilisation are associated with inflammation and cellular communication.

Plaque formation	Plaque destabilisation	Plaque rupture
Vascular risk markers	**Inflammatory markers**	**Cardiac ischemia**
Cholesterol*, HDL*, LDL*, IDL,	C-reactive protein*	Ischaemia-modified albumin
VLDL, non-HDL cholesterol*	Pentraxin 3	Whole blood choline
Cholesterol:HDL*	Oxidised LDL	Unbound free fatty acids
Apolipoprotein A1*	Malondialdehyde	
Apolipoprotein B100*	Myeloperoxidase	
Lp(a) *	Isoprostanes	
Homocysteine*	Xanthine oxidase	
Metabolic markers	**Cytokines**	**Cytosolic proteins**
Albumin*	Tumour necrosis factor alpha	CK-MB*
Insulin*	Interleukin 6	Myoglobin*
Ghrelin	Osteoprotegerin	Heart-type fatty acid-binding protein
Leptin		
Adiponectin		
Resistin		
	Chemokines	**Structural proteins**
	Monocyte chemoattractant factor	Cardiac troponin T*
		Cardiac troponin I*
		Myosin light chain
	Adhesion molecules	**Extracellular matrix turnover and remodelling**
	CD40 ligand	Matrix metalloproteinases (MMP)
	P selectin	Tissue inhibitors of MMP
	E selectin	Procollagen III aminopeptide
	L selectin	Procollagen type 1 COOH-terminal peptide
	Intercellular adhesion molecule-1	Procollagen type 1 NH_2-terminal peptide
	Vascular cell adhesion molecule-1	Basement membrane laminin
	Vascular endothelial growth factor	Tenascin C
		Galectin-3*
	Placental growth factor	
	Hepatic growth factor	
	Endothelial growth factor	
		Biomechanical strain
		Atrial natriuretic peptide
		ProB-type natriuretic peptide*
		B-type natriuretic peptide*
		Interleukin 33/ST 2

Plaque formation	Plaque destabilisation	Plaque rupture
		Growth differentiation factor 15
		Neurohormonal activation
		Aldosterone*
		Copeptin (ADH)
		Adrenomedullin
		Apelin
		Endothelin
		Relaxin
		Urotensin

*Those in routine clinical use.

Table 3. Cardiovascular biomarkers for detection of the cardiovascular disease spectrum categorised into those that detect plaque formation, plaque destabilisation and plaque rupture.

When patients develop symptoms of chest pain, there are biomarkers available to establish a diagnosis of acute plaque rupture. In those who survive AMI and develop chronic heart failure, natriuretic peptides are used for diagnosis and more importantly monitoring of treatment response.

3. Methodology for measurement of cardiac biomarkers

POCT in general costs more per test than that for centralised laboratory diagnostics. Costs are associated with utilising more hardware per test. Single assay cartridges are often used and dedicated instruments are required for detection. Conversely, large platform analysers utilise common detection methods for a number of specific tests and use reagent packs of 100 tests or more. Cost is also proportionate to volume of tests. An instrument, for example, that produces only four cholesterol tests an hour is not suitable for a large routine laboratory setting, where workload for cholesterol determination runs into the hundreds on a daily basis.

Biomarkers produced upstream of plaque rupture and necrosis are associated with assessment of cardiovascular risk. Their primary utility is in low-risk ambulatory patients presenting to the primary care setting. There is no need for urgency in obtaining such results as the clinical presentation is not acute. Similarly, for patients with established Chronic Heart Failure (CHF) managed in primary care, STAT analysis of natriuretic peptides is not warranted. While POCT exist for the determination of high-sensitivity C-reactive protein (hs-CRP) and for B-type natriuretic peptide (BNP) and its NT-pro form (NTproBNP), their use has declined in popularity with the emergence of large high throughput analysers offering similar TAT, at relatively cheaper cost.

Many National and International societies have adopted a TAT of <60 min for cardiac biomarkers. In emergency departments with rapid chest pain protocols, a 30 min TAT is desirable. Centralised pathology provision is possible with pneumatic air tube delivery of samples, STAT processing of samples and host communication with instruments to prioritize samples for 'urgent' analysis over more routine tests that could be performed later. A study in the USA of 159 hospitals, which audited 7020 cTn and 4368 CK-MB determinations, demonstrated TAT of 90 min for cardiac biomarkers [23].

Due to patents, a single manufacturer (Roche Diagnostics) produces assays for cTnT on both large-scale immunoassay analysers and at the point of care. Cardiac troponin I, however, is unlicensed and currently not standardised. A multitude of *in vitro* diagnostic manufacturers produce cTnI methods for both POCT and centralised laboratories. An in-depth review of the measurement of cTn has been published previously [24].

3.1. Point of care testing for cardiac troponin

A number of manufacturers produce POCT cartridges as 'strip tests', which are quantitative methods. These are akin to those used in pregnancy. The rapid stick tests provide a visual detection line to determine a positive result (**Figure 4**) but do not quantify the amount of protein present in the sample. The principle is immunochromatographic lateral flow technology and is common to all strip tests. Fundamentally they work in three steps:

1. *Sample application and separation:* Normally, anticoagulated whole blood is used for POCT to negate the need for clotting and centrifugation. The test actually takes place in the plasma component and requires separation of red blood cells by a capture fleece allowing the plasma to travel in the direction of flow by simple diffusion or by capillary flow in a lumen.

2. *Immunoreactive step:* Antibodies (Ab) against the protein of interest are immobilised on the test strip, which is often made of nitrocellulose. The plasma sample causes mobilisation of the antibodies from the nitrocellulose strip. The sample containing the protein (antigen) of interest combines with the capture and detection antibody to form an Ab-Antigen complex. The detection Ab reacts with a colour-producing substance such as the streptavidin-biotin combination.

3. *Detection step:* The intensity of the colour line produced is proportional to the amount of protein present in the sample. However, it is near impossible to determine differences in intensity with the naked eye.

The vast majority of the strip tests are not validated by the Food and Drug Administration (FDA) or CE marked for European *in vitro* diagnostic use. They are relatively cheap and of benefit in the Developing world, where cost to by technologically advanced readers and the need for power resources are simply not available or cost effective.

In the simulation in **Figure 4**, of note is the internal quality control. As each cartridge is effectively a single run, quality control of a reagent batch or lot number cannot guarantee validity of each individual test cartridge. In the scenario depicted in **Figure 4B–D**, all control lines are present, indicating that each test strip is valid. If a positive line occurs for any of the protein markers in the absence of a control line, the cartridge is not valid and should be voided. The sample should then be repeated on a fresh cartridge.

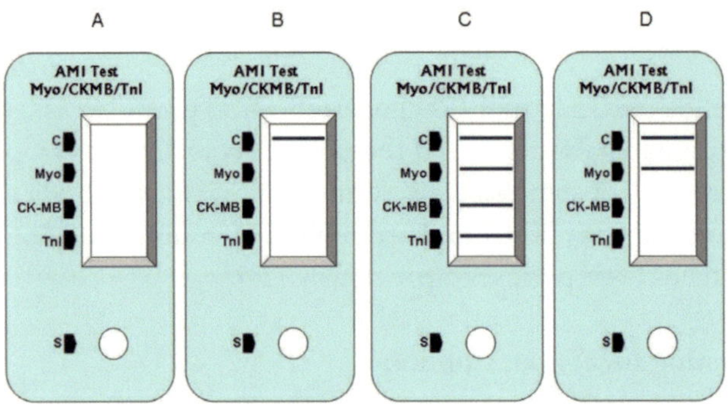

Figure 4. Simulation of a qualitative strip test for a triple panel of cardiac markers. (A) Sample of blood is placed in well at position S. (B) A control line (internal quality control) appears at C to indicate the test strip is valid. (C) A valid test strip positive for myoglobin, CK-MB and cTnI. (D) A valid test strip positive for myoglobin but negative for CK-MB and cTnI.

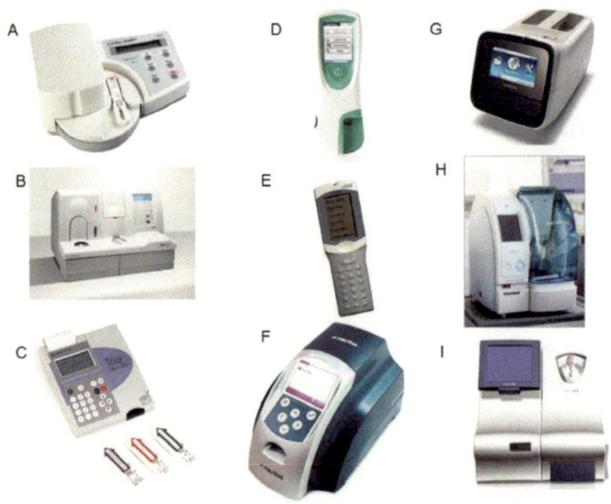

Figure 5. A variety of POCT platforms. (A) Cardiac Reader, Roche Diagnostics; (B) Stratus CS, Siemens Healthcare; (C) Triage, Alere; (D) Cobas h232, Roche Diagnostics; (E) iSTAT, Abbott Laboratories; (F) Meritas, Trinity Biotech; (G) LABGEOIB10, Samsung; (H) PATHFAST, Mitsubishi Chemical Europe and (I) AQT90, Radiometer.

There are a number of portable readers (**Figure 5**) that complement the strip technology in order to quantify the concentration of cTn in the sample. These include the Cardiac Reader and the newer Cobas h232 for cTnT from Roche Diagnostics; the Triage meter for cTnI and BNP (Alere); the Stratus CS for cTnI, myoglobin, CK-MB and NTproBNP, D-dimer and hs-CRP (Siemens Healthcare Diagnostics); the Pathfast for cTnI, myoglobin and CK-MB (Mitsubishi Chemical); the iSTAT for cTnI, CK-MB and BNP (Abbott Laboratories) and the AQT90 flex for cTnT, cTnI, CK-MB, myoglobin, NTproBNP, CRP and D-dimer (Radiometer).

The assay performance characteristics of the cTn POCT reader assays are given in **Table 4**. Since 1979, the WHO criterion for the diagnosis of AMI was the gold standard definition. This was based on the utility of CK-MB measurement, at five times the upper limit of normal. With the advent of cTn assays, which were, in their infancy, rather analytically insensitive, the equivalent value of cTn was adopted as the appropriate cut-off to define AMI. For cTnT, this was 0.1 μg/L. Originally, the cardiac reader reported cTnT values in the range 0.1–50 μg/L. Samples with values below 0.1 μg/L were reported as <0.1 μg/L. The equivalent laboratory-based assay underwent a number of developments to improve analytical performance. The third generation cTnT assay reported to 0.01 μg/L and the clinical cut-off value was 0.03 μg/L. This is lower than that reported by the Cardiac reader and samples in the range 0.03–0.09 μg/L would have been deemed positive in the centralised laboratory and negative by the Cardiac Reader.

Manufacturer/instrument /assay	Capture antibody epitope (aa residues)	Detection antibody epitope (aa residues)	Detection antibody tag
Abbott Laboratories i-STAT	41–49, 88–91	28–39, 62–78	ALP
Inverness Biosite Triage	NA	27–40	Fluorophore
Mitsubishi Chemical PATHFAST	41–49	71–116, 163–209	ALP
Radiometer AQT90	41–49, 190–196	137–149	Europium
Response Biomedical RAMP	85–92	26–38	Fluorophore
Roche Cardiac Reader cTnT	125–131	136–147	Gold particles
Siemens Stratus CS	27–32	41–56	ALP

aa, amino acid; ALP, alkaline phosphatase.

Table 4. POCT assay characteristics for cardiac troponin measurement.

3.2. Clinical application of POCT cardiac troponin testing

If the turnaround time cannot be realised by the central laboratory, POCT at satellite locations or near the patient can improve the diagnostic decision process. A number of studies have demonstrated a sufficient reduction in turnaround time from 87 to 25 min in order to meet international guidelines [11, 25–27]. The biggest disadvantage to POCT is the cost per assay compared to that of the central laboratory, making POCT an expensive alternative.

Multiple cardiac biomarker measurements have been advocated for the early diagnosis of AMI. The utility is based on the presence of a lag period in cardiac necrosis. Initially, when cells die, elevation of cTn may not be detectable until a significant amount of cellular damage has occurred. In the initial 3 h from chest pain onset, the measurement of myoglobin or the CK-MB may be appropriate especially in the point of care setting and a protocol based on triple cardiac marker testing has been suggested [27] and validated [28]. However, the introduction of assays in the centralised laboratory capable of measuring troponin concentrations within the reference interval [29] and the detection of very early rises in cTn [30, 31] in the initial 3 h from presentation challenges this concept.

To date, there have been four randomised control trials of point of care testing [11, 32–34]. Two studies report outcomes [11, 34] with no difference in the number of adverse events in patients randomised to either POCT or central pathology laboratory testing. One study reported diagnostic accuracy, observing that POCT and central laboratory testing were equivalent [11]. In this study, a POCT cTnT method with the same decision limit as that in use by the central laboratory method of 0.1 μg/L. Although appropriate at the time of the study, the 0.1 μg/L decision limit is now considered too high for centralised cTnT determination. Further studies are required to assess the utility of POCT for cardiac troponin in comparison to high-sensitive methodology available in the central laboratory.

In the recent multicentre, Randomised Assessment of Treatment, using Panel Assay of Cardiac Markers (RATPAC) study performed in the UK, Goodacre et al. demonstrated that POCT increases successful discharge home of patients within 4 h of attendance and significantly reduced the median length of stay (8.8 h in POCT arm compared to 14.2 h in the central lab testing arm). There was no effect in overall bed use [35]. The use of POCT was associated with higher cost in the ED, coronary care and increased cardiac intervention costs but overall lower general inpatient costs [36].

3.3. POCT cardiac troponin in the pre-hospital setting

There are very limited data using point of care testing (POCT) for cTn in the pre-hospital setting. The majority utilised the initial rapid Trop T assay from Roche Diagnostics [37–39], which was far less sensitive than we are used to in current laboratory diagnostics. The cut-off for AMI was 0.1 μg/L which equates to 100 ng/L in new units. By contrast, the current hs-cTnT assay has a 99th percentile cut-off value of 14 ng/L. There are even less published data using POCT cTnI [40–42].

What is important to remember is that the current POCT technology for cTn is not suitably analytically sensitive enough when compared to laboratory-based immunoassay. To this end, they are reliable as rule in tests if patients are positive for cTn; however, their role as a rule out marker is questionable due to the equivalent high cut-off values employed.

In urban areas, where patients receive rapid response to emergency calls within minutes with subsequent rapid transfer, the value of POCT is questionable. However, if a suitable sensitive POCT could be developed, this may have major benefit in rural areas, where patients can be triaged to appropriate cardiac centres that offer immediate primary coronary interventional surgery. Furthermore, it is not common practice to draw venous blood samples in the pre-hospital setting by paramedical staff. There are a number of companies that are investing in new technology with the hope of delivering a sensitive POCT troponin test with the added benefit of possibly using finger-prick testing rather than venepuncture. The Samsung device

1B10 cTnI assay has been studied in the Scottish Ambulance Service. The pilot study demonstrated that patients with non-ST segment elevation myocardial infarction who demonstrated elevated cTnI in the pre-hospital setting benefited from disposition triage similar to those with ECG changes indicative of an ST elevation AMI. The pre-hospital cTnI measurement gives a documented actual time zero from pain up to 2 h earlier than in-hospital testing, leading to a reduction in time to second measurement if the initial sample was negative or detectable but below the 99th percentile cut-off for positive [43].

The demand for POCT by finger-prick testing is attractive across many disciplines and would be of benefit for self-monitoring at home by patients. This is already in common practice for diabetic patients but has practical implications for others such as those with CHF. However, a recent publication by Bond and Richards-Kortum has demonstrated vast differences in haematological parameters when using capillary blood sampling. The coefficient of variation for platelets was 19% when using capillary blood compared to 4–5% when using venous blood samples. Higher CVs were also obtained from lymphocytes, granulocytes and haemoglobin determination [44].

4. Conclusion

Point of care testing for cardiac biomarkers is only practical for the measurement of acute biomarkers of necrosis such as the cardiac troponins. Risk markers are not required urgently and therefore can be performed in a more cost-effective manner by centralised laboratory testing. Recent advances in centralised laboratory testing have resulted in more sensitive methods available with improved TAT. These cannot be met by the current POCT technology. Alternative detection methodologies are required for providing robust low concentration analysis of proteins in small sample volumes at relatively cheap cost.

5. Executive summary

- Cardiac disease is the largest cause of morbidity and mortality in the world.
- Cardiac troponins T and I are considered the gold standard diagnostic test for the detection of acute coronary syndromes.
- POCT for risk markers, such as lipids and C-reactive protein, is not cost effective.
- POCT technology for cTnT and cTnI cannot meet the current analytical performance of centralised laboratory testing.
- Novel technology is required to make POCT more sensitive analytically, which will have a major impact on clinical performance.

Author details

David C. Gaze*

Address all correspondence to: david.gaze@stgeorges.nhs.uk

Department of Chemical Pathology Clinical Blood Sciences, St George's Healthcare NHS Trust, London, United Kingdom

References

[1] Price CP. Point-of-care testing, 2nd edn. Washington DC, USA: AACC Press, 2004.

[2] Jacobs E, Nowakowski M, Colman N. Performance of Gem Premier blood gas/ electrolyte analyzer evaluated. *Clin Chem*. 1993;39:1890–1893.

[3] Lindemans J, Hoefkens P, Van Kessel AL et al. Portable blood gas and electrolyte analyzer evaluated in a multiinstitutional study. *Clin Chem*. 1999;45:111–117.

[4] Wong RJ, Mahoney JJ, Van Kessel AL. Evaluation of the Ciba Corning 840 blood gas analyzer. *Respir Care*. 1995;40:638–643.

[5] Wong RJ, Mahoney JJ, Harvey JA et al. StatPal II pH and Blood Gas Analysis System evaluated. *Clin Chem*. 1994;40:124–129.

[6] Gregory LC, Duh SH, Christenson RH. Eight compact analysis systems evaluated for measuring total cholesterol. *Clin Chem*. 1994;40:579–585.

[7] Bereznicki LR, Jackson SL, Peterson GM et al. Accuracy and clinical utility of the CoaguChek XS portable international normalised ratio monitor in a pilot study of warfarin home-monitoring. *J Clin Pathol*. 2007;60:311–314.

[8] Despotis GJ, Santoro SA, Spitznagel E et al. Prospective evaluation and clinical utility of on-site monitoring of coagulation in patients undergoing cardiac operation. *J Thorac Cardiovasc Surg*. 1994;107:271–279.

[9] Tsai WW, Nash DB, Seamonds B et al. Point-of-care versus central laboratory testing: an economic analysis in an academic medical center. *Clin Ther*. 1994;16:898–910.

[10] Kilgore ML, Steindel SJ, Smith JA. Evaluating stat testing options in an academic health center: therapeutic turnaround time and staff satisfaction. *Clin Chem*. 1998;44:1597–1603.

[11] Collinson PO, John C, Lynch S et al. A prospective randomized controlled trial of point-of-care testing on the coronary care unit. *Ann Clin Biochem*. 2004;41:397–404.

[12] Parvin CA, Lo SF, Deuser SM et al. Impact of point-of-care testing on patients' length of stay in a large emergency department. *Clin Chem*. 1996;42:711–717.

[13] Kendall J, Reeves B, Clancy M. Point of care testing: randomised controlled trial of clinical outcome. *BMJ*. 1998;316:1052–1057.

[14] Collinson PO, Gaze DC, Bainbridge K et al. Utility of admission cardiac troponin and "Ischemia Modified Albumin" measurements for rapid evaluation and rule out of suspected acute myocardial infarction in the emergency department. *Emerg Med J*. 2006;23:256–261.

[15] Collinson PO, Gaze DC. Ischaemia-modified albumin: clinical utility and pitfalls in measurement. *J Clin Pathol*. 2008;61:1025–1028.

[16] Pope JH, Aufderheide TP, Ruthazer R et al. Missed diagnoses of acute cardiac ischemia in the emergency department. *N Engl J Med*. 2000;342:1163–1170.

[17] Collinson PO, Premachandram S, Hashemi K. Prospective audit of incidence of prognostically important myocardial damage in patients discharged from emergency department. *BMJ*. 2000;320:1702–1705.

[18] Pozen MW, D'Agostino RB, Selker HP et al. A predictive instrument to improve coronary-care-unit admission practices in acute ischemic heart disease. A prospective multicenter clinical trial. *N Engl J Med*. 1984;310:1273–1278.

[19] de Dombal FT, Clamp SE, Softley A et al. Prediction of individual patient prognosis: value of computer-aided systems. *Med Decis Making*. 1986;6:18–22.

[20] Goldman L, Cook EF, Brand DA et al. A computer protocol to predict myocardial infarction in emergency department patients with chest pain. *N Engl J Med*. 1988;318:797–803.

[21] Willems JL, Willems RJ, Bijnens I et al. Value of electrocardiographic scoring systems for the assessment of thrombolytic therapy in acute myocardial infarction. The European Cooperative Study Group for Recombinant Tissue Type Plasminogen Activator. *Eur Heart J*. 1991;12:378–388.

[22] Gaze DC, Collinson PO. Cardiac troponins as biomarkers of drug- and toxin-induced cardiac toxicity and cardioprotection. *Expert Opin Drug Metab Toxicol*. 2005;1:715–725.

[23] Novis DA, Jones BA, Dale JC et al. Biochemical markers of myocardial injury test turnaround time: a College of American Pathologists Q-Probes study of 7020 troponin and 4368 creatine kinase-MB determinations in 159 institutions. *Arch Pathol Lab Med*. 2004;128:158–164.

[24] Collinson PO, Boa FG, Gaze DC. Measurement of cardiac troponins. *Ann Clin Biochem*. 2001;38:423–449.

[25] Caragher TE, Fernandez BB, Jacobs FL et al. Evaluation of quantitative cardiac biomarker point-of-care testing in the emergency department. *J Emerg Med*. 2002;22:1–7.

[26] Lee-Lewandrowski E, Corboy D, Lewandrowski K et al. Implementation of a point-of-care satellite laboratory in the emergency department of an academic medical center. Impact on test turnaround time and patient emergency department length of stay. *Arch Pathol Lab Med*. 2003;127:456–460.

[27] McCord J, Nowak RM, McCullough PA et al. Ninety-minute exclusion of acute myocardial infarction by use of quantitative point-of-care testing of myoglobin and troponin I. *Circulation*. 2001;104:1483–1488.

[28] Ng SM, Krishnaswamy P, Morrisey R et al. Mitigation of the clinical significance of spurious elevations of cardiac troponin I in settings of coronary ischemia using serial testing of multiple cardiac markers. *Am J Cardiol*. 2001;87:994–999.

[29] Collinson PO, Clifford-Mobley O, Gaze D et al. Assay imprecision and 99th-percentile reference value of a high-sensitivity cardiac troponin I assay. *Clin Chem*. 2009;55:1433–1434.

[30] Apple FS. A new season for cardiac troponin assays: it's time to keep a scorecard. *Clin Chem*. 2009;55:1303–1306.

[31] Kavsak PA, McQueen MJ. Sensitive and high sensitivity cardiac troponin I concentrations in the Heart Outcomes Prevention Evaluation (HOPE) study—a high risk population. *Clin Chim Acta*. 2010;411:1832.

[32] Loten C, Attia J, Hullick C et al. Point of care troponin decreases time in the emergency department for patients with possible acute coronary syndrome: a randomised controlled trial. *Emerg Med J*. 2010;27:194–198.

[33] Ryan RJ, Lindsell CJ, Hollander JE et al. A multicenter randomized controlled trial comparing central laboratory and point-of-care cardiac marker testing strategies: the Disposition Impacted by Serial Point of Care Markers in Acute Coronary Syndromes (DISPO-ACS) trial. *Ann Emerg Med*. 2009;53:321–328.

[34] Renaud B, Maison P, Ngako A et al. Impact of point-of-care testing in the emergency department evaluation and treatment of patients with suspected acute coronary syndromes. *Acad Emerg Med*. 2008;15:216–224.

[35] Goodacre SW, Bradburn M, Cross E et al. The Randomised Assessment of Treatment using Panel Assay of Cardiac Markers (RATPAC) trial: a randomised controlled trial of point-of-care cardiac markers in the emergency department. *Heart*. 2011;97:190–196.

[36] Fitzgerald P, Goodacre SW, Cross E et al. Cost-effectiveness of point-of-care biomarker assessment for suspected myocardial infarction: the randomized assessment of treatment using panel assay of cardiac markers (RATPAC) trial. *Acad Emerg Med*. 2011;18:488–495.

[37] Newman J, Aulick N, Cheng T et al. Prehospital identification of acute coronary ischemia using a troponin T rapid assay. *Prehosp Emerg Care*. 1999;3:97–101.

[38] Schuchert A, Hamm C, Scholz J et al. Prehospital testing for troponin T in patients with suspected acute myocardial infarction. *Am Heart J*. 1999;138:45–48.

[39] Sorensen JT, Terkelsen CJ, Steengaard C et al. Prehospital troponin T testing in the diagnosis and triage of patients with suspected acute myocardial infarction. *Am J Cardiol*. 2011;107:1436–1440.

[40] Dumas F, Manzo-Silberman S, Fichet J et al. Can early cardiac troponin I measurement help to predict recent coronary occlusion in out-of-hospital cardiac arrest survivors? *Crit Care Med*. 2012;40:1777–1784.

[41] Venturini JM, Stake CE, Cichon ME. Prehospital point-of-care testing for troponin: are the results reliable? *Prehosp Emerg Care*. 2013;17:88–91.

[42] Ezekowitz JA, Welsh RC, Weiss D et al. Providing Rapid Out of Hospital Acute Cardiovascular Treatment 4 (PROACT-4). *J Am Heart Assoc*. 2015;4.

[43] Scotland S, Lunts P, Nicoll G, Barclay K, Baxter C, Archibald I, Miller G, Bluestein BI, Brennan E, Kim D, Grant J, Dean K. Evaluation of point of care (POC) Prehospital testing for troponin I (cTnI) while in Hospital Transit via the Scottish Ambulance Service (SAS)—a Preliminary Study using the Samsung LABGEOIB10 Analyzer. Clin Chem. 2013;59(10): A182.

[44] Bond MM, Richards-Kortum RR. Drop-to-drop variation in the cellular components of fingerprick blood: implications for point-of-care diagnostic development. *Am J Clin Pathol*. 2015;144:885–894.

Section 3

RDTs' in Diagnosis of Paediatric Oncology

Chapter 3

Alpha-Fetoprotein in Malignant Pediatric Conditions

Lisa Van Houwelingen and John A. Sandoval

Additional information is available at the end of the chapter

http://dx.doi.org/10.5772/63911

Abstract

Abnormal serum α-fetoprotein (AFP) levels are frequently observed in common disorders such as spina bifida or Down's syndrome in the fetus and cancer in children and adults. The focus of this chapter summarizes on the role of serum α-fetoprotein (AFP) as a useful biomarker in malignant pediatric tumors. The fetal yolk sac and liver generate high levels of AFP during gestation and decline over the next 12 months of infancy, and only trace amounts are detected in childhood. As a result, persistent elevation of AFP correlates with a number of select pediatric malignant conditions. Serum AFP is overexpressed in a considerable fraction of germ cell tumors (GCTs), hepatoblastoma (HB), and hepatocellular carcinoma (HCC). We provide the reader with a review of AFP as a useful specific marker for the diagnosis, management, and follow-up in select pediatric cancers.

Keywords: α-fetoprotein, oncofetal protein, germ cell tumors, hepatoblastoma, hepatocellular carcinoma

1. Introduction

The accurate diagnosis of pediatric solid tumors and the timely recognition of disease recurrence involve the combination of clinical suspicion, imaging techniques, tissue biopsy, and serum tumor markers. Traditional cancer biomarkers are biologically measured substances that are expressed by malignant tissues, or generated by the host in response to the tumor and aid the clinician in diagnosis, staging, assessing response to treatment, and detecting disease recurrence [1]. Tumor markers can be measured in the blood, cerebrospinal fluid, or serous effusions. In general, elevated levels of these biomarkers have been implicated as playing an important role in different types of cancer, and some play a significant role as prognostic indicators [2].

Bergstrand and Czar first identified α-fetoprotein (AFP) in human fetuses in 1956 [3]. Characterized as a glycoprotein that is normally produced during gestation by the yolk sac and the liver during fetal life, AFP is highly elevated in the circulation of newborns, and concentration decreases (half-life, 5 days) to 10–20 μg/L during the first 12 months of infant life [4]. A major mammalian oncofetal protein, AFP is a member of the albuminoid gene superfamily, which consists of AFP, serum albumin, vitamin D-binding protein, and alpha-albumin (afamin) on chromosome 4. AFP is found in monomeric as well as in dimeric and trimeric forms, and binds copper, nickel, fatty acids, and bilirubin [5]. In normal fetuses, AFP binds the hormone estradiol. Altered serum AFP levels have been observed concurrent with aberrant growth manifestation in some birth defects (increased in open neural tube defects, and omphalocele and decreased in Down syndrome) and a subset of endodermal-derived malignancies, most frequently hepatoblastoma (HB), hepatocellular carcinoma (HCC), and germ cell tumors (GCTs), some esophageal and pancreatic carcinomas, and also some benign conditions, particularly those associated with liver damage and regeneration [6]. Given that age-dependent changes in serum AFP levels occur, the consideration of infants' ages while interpreting AFP levels should be underscored. AFP reaches its peak concentration at approximately 12–14 weeks of gestation as this fetal protein is initially synthesized in the yolk sac and then is generated by hepatocytes and gastrointestinal mucosa during embryogenesis. Levels subsequently decline and reach a normal concentration at 8–12 months of age [7]. Because serum AFP concentrations are highly elevated in neonates and exceedingly high levels can be observed in premature infants, AFP levels should be interpreted based on the infant's age and gestational period; normal median levels in term neonates are 41,687 l g/L, and preterm infants, 158,125 l g/L [8].

Due to the age-related changes in AFP values, and the fact that this biomarker is a tumor-associated, not tumor-specific protein, elevation of AFP levels alone does not allow for the diagnosis of malignancy. Additional workup and evaluation including pathologic diagnosis, imaging, and exclusion of other conditions associated with elevations of AFP must compliment tumor marker evaluation. An AFP serum level above 500 μg/L is rarely associated with a benign diagnosis [2].

2. Germ cell tumors

As approximately 50% of GCTs are benign (pure mature teratoma) and do not secrete AFP, the exact incidence of pediatric GCTs is not precisely known. Malignant GCTs account for 3% of all childhood cancers, with 350 new pediatric germ cell tumors diagnosed each year. These tumors develop from variations in normal differentiation (gonadal GCT) and/or aberrant migration (extragonadal GCT) of primordial germ cells. Extragonadal GCTs occur in a variety of midline locations (retroperitoneal, genital, or cranial) but most affect the mediastinum and the sacrococcygeal region. Two groups of GCTs are morphologically divided into seminomas and non-seminomatous germ cell tumors (NSGCTs). Most NSGCTs are a mixture of histologies such as embryonal, choriocarcinomas, teratomas, and yolk sac tumors (YSTs).

Malignant GCTs with yolk sac tumor differentiation are readily characterized with AFP secretion [2]. While predicting behavior in GCT can be confusing secondary to varying factors such as patient age, anatomic site, histologic subtype, and clinical stage, serum levels of AFP are well known in its utility as a noninvasive diagnostic indicator of GCT with yolk sac component [9]. This marker is well validated in its utility as a diagnostic indicator, staging, monitoring of therapeutic response, and subsequent follow-up [10]. In infants and adolescents who are without underlying hepatic disease, a significant elevation of AFP represents a predominant YST component and precludes the diagnosis of a pure mature teratoma or seminoma [1].

The diagnosis of malignant germ cell tumor involves the evaluation of serum AFP in conjunction with the review of histopathology and diagnostic imaging. At times, and often due to sampling error, the pathology may fail to identify a yolk sac component even when the serum AFP is elevated. This is particularly true for intracranial GCT where only limited tissue biopsies are possible [2, 11, 12].

The clinical use of AFP extends beyond initial diagnosis. Tumor marker follow-up examination is also performed during neo-adjuvant chemotherapy to assess for tumor response to therapy. A failure of AFP to decline during chemotherapy may cause clinicians to reevaluate the need for earlier surgical intervention or adjustment of chemotherapy regimen. Prognostic subgroups have been defined based on the ability to evaluate tumor chemotherapy response. For instance, the International Germ Cell Classification Consensus (IGCCC) divides adults into three prognostic groups: good, intermediate, and poor based on the presence of primary tumor, non-pulmonary metastases, and level of tumor biomarkers [10]. Risk-group stratification allows for individual treatment tailoring as well as comparison of results across populations of similarly defined patients and ultimately the collaboration of international clinical trials [13]. This has not yet translated to pediatric oncology as pediatric GCTs are typically divided into risk groups according to stage, histologic grade, and site (gonadal vs. extragonadal). Serum markers have not contributed to risk stratification. The importance of age and level of AFP at diagnosis have varied among studies. A number of groups, including the Children's Cancer and Leukemia Group (CCLG), the French Society of Pediatric Oncology, and Children's Oncology Group (COG), have previously identified serum AFP (>10,000 ng/mL) as a prognostic factor [13–15]. An investigation by the Children's Oncology Group (COG) and the CCLG compared the application of the adult IGCC system to pediatric malignant NSGCT by pooling 25 years worth of clinical trial results. The groups aimed to determine if the tumor biomarker criteria developed in adults would be prognostic among pediatric patients and they also queried whether tumor biomarker data may be relevant in pediatric risk stratification. The results of the study determined that AFP was not prognostic of outcome in pediatric patients, and therefore the utility of AFP in risk stratification in pediatric malignant GCT remains unsettled [16].

Another rare finding while on neo-adjuvant chemotherapy is the growing teratoma syndrome in which a patient with a mixed GCT demonstrates radiographic progression of disease with a reduction of tumor marker. The rationale for continued growth of the tumor is based on the observation that progressive proliferation of the mature or immature components of the teratoma occurs while the YST component responds to chemotherapy. In this case, prompt surgical excision of the tumor is generally recommended [17, 18].

A final use of AFP as a tumor marker is found following completion of therapy (surgery, chemotherapy, or combination) to assess for the recurrence of disease. The goal after therapy is to have normalization of serum AFP. Tumor recurrence is demonstrated by an abrupt elevation of the AFP level. Yolk sac tumors and mixed germ cell tumors require close follow-up with serial AFP level monitoring as part of the surveillance strategy for this patient population.

3. Hepatoblastoma and hepatocellular carcinoma

Approximately 100–150 new cases of primary liver malignancies are diagnosed annually in the USA and represent for slightly more than 1% of all pediatric tumors [19]. Hepatoblastoma (HB), hepatocellular carcinoma (HCC), sarcomas, germ cell tumors, and rhabdoid tumors constitute the spectrum of malignant liver tumors seen in children. The majority of these are embryonal HB, which accounts for over half (66%) of malignant hepatic neoplasms.

Serum AFP levels are an important tumor marker for HB and HCC. In addition, serum AFP levels may also be elevated in other nonmalignant states such as mesenchymal hamartoma, infantile hepatic hemangioendothelioma, cirrhosis, viral and chronic active hepatitis, tyrosinemia, ulcerative colitis, and in various immune-deficiency conditions [20, 21].

Most children with HB have extremely elevated serum AFP levels (up to 100,000 ± 1,000,000 times the normal value (<10 ng/mL)), but roughly 5–10% of patients have unexpectedly low or even normal AFP levels [22]. For HB, serum AFP level is a required diagnostic test, given the correlation between AFP level and tumor burden. Additionally, serial determinations of AFP determine the effectiveness of therapy as AFP concentrations decline to normal levels with effective therapy and persistently elevated levels suggest residual disease. The half-life of the circulating oncoprotein in the bloodstream is between 4 and 9 days, and levels usually return to the normal range (<10 ng/mL) by 4 ± 6 weeks of complete resection [23, 24]. Rising levels following surgery suggest disease progression, recurrence, incomplete tumor resection, or metastases.

Serum AFP is also used as a screening tool to detect the development of HB in children with Beckwith-Wiedemann syndrome (BWS) or isolated hemihyperplasia (HH). The development of HB in these cancer predisposition syndromes has been observed in 1–3% of patients with BWS and HH. Improved survival is dependent on early detection. This can be inferred by the improved prognosis of early stage (stage I and II) HB as compared to late stage (stage III and IV) tumors: 91% of 5-year event-free survival vs. 25–64% of 5-year event-free survival, respectively. This is accomplished by routine screening with hepatic ultrasound and serum AFP at 3-month intervals up to the age of 4 years [25].

A final use of serum AFP in children with HB is its use in prognostication. Although complete surgical resection in HB is the best predictor of survival, more than half of children initially present with advanced unresectable disease (stage III or IV, North American Staging System). In an effort to achieve cytoreduction and improved resectability, children with up-front unresectable HB receive neo-adjuvant cisplatin-based chemotherapy [26]. HB patients who are poor responders to induction therapy (as demonstrated by persistently elevated AFP levels) have been shown to have a significantly worse outcome [23]. In fact, the strongest predictor of survival in unresectable or metastatic HB is the timing and significance of the AFP level change during neo-adjuvant chemotherapy administration. A large early decrease in AFP level correlates with the best outcome. It has been further suggested that monitoring the changes in AFP during neo-adjuvant chemotherapy may help identify poor responders and, in those patients, we should consider a change in therapeutic approach [27].

Another poor predictor of survival is low serum AFP at diagnosis. Although most patients present with elevated levels, serum AFP is low or normal in approximately 5–10% of cases. Children with HB and low AFP level at diagnosis have been identified as a high-risk group. This group of patients will generally present with more advanced disease at diagnosis and have a high degree of treatment failure [28].

HB can also be linked with the abnormal secretion of peptide hormones and other proteins. Marked thrombocytosis secondary to the release of tumor-derived elements with growth factors, thrombopoietin-like activity, platelet-derived microparticles, components released from bone marrow endothelial cells, and growth-related factors secreted by megakaryocytes can impact these biologic processes [29–31]. Likewise, ectopic beta subunit of human chorionic gonadotropin (βHCG) secretion can lead to precocious puberty in boys (virilizing HB) or a *forme fruste* in girls [32]. Grunewald and scholars reported a case study of a hormonally active HB causing both ectopic adrenocorticotropic hormone (ACTH) syndrome and parathyroid hormone (PTH)-related peptide-induced hypercalcemia [33]. While these paraneoplastic syndromes are not commonly associated to HB, they stress the importance of considering these oncofetal antigens as tumor-associated rather than tumor-specific, and the varied clinical presentations that can pose further diagnostic and therapeutic challenges in HB.

HCC is the second most common hepatic malignancy in children and accounts for less than 0.5% of all pediatric cancer [34]. An estimated 0.5–1.0 cases per million children is the reported relative frequency for HCC [35]. Unlike HB, it is more commonly found in older children and teenagers with underlying liver conditions (Alagille syndrome, viral hepatitis B/C, progressive familial intrahepatic cholestasis, inborn errors of metabolism [tyrosinemia and glycogen storage diseases I–IV]). The 5-year overall survival (OS) rate is 42% for children and adolescents with hepatocellular carcinoma. The use of AFP levels in HCC has been primarily for diagnostic purposes. Most HCCs are associated with elevated levels of AFP. Although not found to be an independent predictor of survival, it has been observed that HCCs with serum AFP of <100 ng/mL at diagnosis tend to have a worse outcome and are frequently observed in the fibrolamellar HCC variant [36]. Serum AFP may also be used for surveillance purposes in the "at-risk" patient. Patients treated for biliary atresia (obstructive cholangiopathy of the newborn) in infancy should be monitored for the development of cirrhosis and subsequently HCC as well as cholangiocarcinoma. This can be accomplished with abdominal ultrasound and serum AFP levels at 6–12-month intervals [37]. Children who are diagnosed with inborn errors of metabolism, congenital malformations, or who have cirrhosis induced by chronic liver disease require screening for the development of HCC.

4. AFP and associated rare pediatric solid cancers

While serum AFP is primarily used in the diagnosis and management of GCT (with yolk sac component), HB, and HCC, elevated levels have also been found in select cases of nephroblastoma (Wilms tumor, WT) and pancreatoblastoma (PB). For example, Roth and colleagues first described WT presenting with elevated serum AFP [38]. Since this initial description, only four other WT cases have been documented with histologically classic type WT and elevated AFP [39–41]. More notably, elevated AFP is seen in the teratoid WT, in which more than 50% of the tumor is composed of teratoid elements [42]. Nevertheless, due to the extremely rare occurrence, serum AFP is not a typical tumor marker for pediatric renal tumors.

PB is a rare childhood malignancy with only 62 cases reported in the literature [43]. It has been described as an embryonal hamartomatous neoplasm arising from multipotential stem cells [44]. Typically presenting as an abdominal mass with progressive jaundice, PB has been associated with an elevated serum AFP at diagnosis in 25% of the described cases. While clinically affiliated with a prolonged, indolent course with favorable outcomes, serum AFP may contribute to the diagnosis and monitoring of therapy for PB [45].

5. Conclusion

Although AFP is a well-known classical serum biomarker that can assist with diagnosis of certain malignant solid tumors in children, it remains limited in sensitivity and specificity [46]. Other promising biomarkers for tumor diagnosis, especially GCT, include microRNAs (miRNAs), which are short nucleic acid molecules synthesized in the cellular nucleus. miRNAs modify posttranscriptional gene activity by targeting mRNA molecules. Once released from the nucleus, miRNAs can enter almost all biological fluids (e.g., serum, saliva, urine, and milk), where they are thought to mediate intercellular communication. After departure from the cell of origin, miRNAs show remarkable stability because of their inclusion in membrane vesicles (exosomes). As a result, blood-based miRNAs show considerable promise for cancer diagnosis and monitoring [47]. miRNAs encoded by the small miR-371-3 cluster that maps to the terminal region of the long arm of chromosome 19 are among the most promising candidates for diagnosing and monitoring malignant GCTs, as these tumors overexpress the miR-371-373 and miR-302/367 clusters, regardless of the age of the patient, the histological subtype of the tumor, or its anatomical site [47]. Murray et al. have reviewed the current understanding of miRNAs and their role in diagnosing and monitoring childhood GCTs [48]. The applicability of miRNAs for the screening and diagnosis to clinical decision-making aids, surveillance biomarkers, or sources of real-time molecular characterization may emerge as the next generation "smart" biomarkers for pediatric solid malignancies.

http://dx.doi.org/10.5772/63911

Author details

Lisa Van Houwelingen[1] and John A. Sandoval[2*]

*Address all correspondence to: john.sandoval@bmg.md

1 St Jude Children's Research Hospital, Memphis, TN, USA

2 Baptist Children's Hospital, Memphis, TN, USA

References

[1] Sandoval, J.A.; Malkas, L.H.; Hickey, R.J. Clinical Significance of Serum Biomarkers in Pediatric Solid Mediastinal and Abdominal Tumors. *Int J Mol Sci* 2012; 13:1126–1153.

[2] Schnieder, D.T.; Calaminus, G.; Gobel, U. Diagnostic Value of Alpha-Fetoprotein and Beta-Human Chorionic Gonadotropin in infancy and Childhood. *Pediatr Hematol Oncol* 2001; 18: 11–26.

[3] Bergstrand C.G.; Czar B. Demonstration of a New Protein Fraction in Serum from the Human Fetus. *Scand J Clin Lab Invest* 1956; 8: 174.

[4] Blohm, M.E.; Vesterling-Horner, D; Calaminus,G; Gobel, U. Alpha 1-Fetoprotein (AFP) Reference Values in Infants up to 2 Years of Age. *Pediatr Hematol Oncol* 1998; 15(2): 135–142.

[5] Aoyagi, Y.; Ikenaka, T.; Ichida, F. alpha-Fetoprotein as a Carrier Protein in Plasma and its Bilirubin-Binding Ability. *Cancer Res* 1979; 39(9):3571–3574.

[6] Marshall, W.; Bangert, S. Clinical Biochemistry: Metabolic and Clinical Aspects. 2nd ed. Philadelphia, PA: Churchill Livingstone, Elsevier; 2008.

[7] Mueller, B.U.; Lopez-Terrada, D., Finegold, M.J. Tumors of the Liver. In *Principles and Practices of Pediatric Oncology*, 5th ed; Pizzo, P., Poplack, D., Eds. Philadelphia, PA: Lippincott Williams & Wilkins., 2006; pp. 887–904.

[8] Wu, J.T.; Book, L.; Sudar, K. Serum alpha-Fetoprotein (AFP) Levels in Normal Infants. *Pediatr Res* 1981; 15: 50–52.

[9] Billmire, D., Vinocur, C., Rescorla, F. et al. Outcome and Staging Evaluation in Malignant Germ Cell Tumors of the Ovary in Children and Adolescents: An Intergroup Study. *J Pediatr Surg* 2004; 39(3): 424–429.

[10] International Germ Cell Cancer Collaborative Group. International Germ Cell Consensus Classification: A Prognostic Factor-based Staging System for Metastatic Germ Cell Cancers. *J Clin Oncol* 1997; 15: 594–603.

[11] Gobel, U.; Calaminus, G.; Engert, J. Teratomas in Infancy and Childhood. *Med Pediatr Oncol* 1998; 31: 8–15.

[12] Harms, D.; Janig, U. Germ Cell Tumors of Childhood: Report of 170 Cases Including 59 Pure and Partial Yolk Sac Tumors. *Virchows Arch A* 1986; 409: 223–239.

[13] Frazier, A.L.; Rumcheva, P.; Olson,T.; Giller, R.; Cushing, B.; Cullen, J.; Marina, N.; London, W.B. Application of the Adult International Germ Cell Classification System to Pediatric Malignant Non-Seminomatous Germ Cell Tumors: A Report from the Children's Oncology Group. *Pediatr Blood Cancer* 2008; 50: 746–751.

[14] Mann, J.R.; Raafat, F.; Robinson, K.; Imerson, J.; Gornall, P.; Sokal, M.; Gray, E.; McKeever, P.; Hale, J.; Bailey, S.; Oakhill, A. The United Kingdom Children's Cancer Study Group's Second Germ Cell Tumor Study: Carboplatin, Etoposide, and Bleomycin are Effective Treatment for Children with Malignant Extracranial Germ Cell Tumors, with Acceptable Toxicity. *J Clin Oncol* 2000; 18: 3809–3818.

[15] Baranzelli, M.C.; Kramar, A.; Bouffet, E.; Quintana, E.; Rubie, H.; Edan, C.; Patte, C. Prognostic Factors in Children with Localized Malignant Nonseminomatous Germ Cell Tumors. *J Clin Oncol* 1999; 17: 1212.

[16] Frazier, A.L.; Hale, J.P.; Rodriguez-Galindo, C.; Dang, H.; Olson, T.; Murray, M.J.; Amatruda, J.F.; Thornton, C.; Arul, G.S.; Billmire, D.; Shaikh,F.; Farzana,P.; Stoneham, S.; Krailo, M.; Nicholso, J.C. Revised Risk Classification for Pediatric Extracranial Germ Cell Tumors Based on 25 Years of Clinical Trial Data From the United Kingdom and United States. *J Clin Oncol* 2015; 33:195–201.

[17] Chen LT, Chen CL, Hwang WS. The growing teratoma syndrome. A case of primary mediastinal nonseminomatous germ cell tumor treated with chemotherapy and radiotherapy. *Chest*. 1990 Jul;98(1):231–3.

[18] Afifi HY, Burt ME. Mediastinal growing teratoma syndrome. *Ann Thorac Surg*. 1997 Aug;64(2):359–62.

[19] Bulterys, M.; Goodman, M.T.; Smith, M.; Buckley, J.D. Hepatic Tumors. In Cancer Incidence, Survival Among Children, Adolescents: United States SEER Program 1975–1995. Available online: http://seer.cancer.gov/publications/childhood/ (access on 12 November 2015).

[20] Urbach, A.H.; Zitelli, B.J.; Blatt, J.; Gartner, J.C.; Malatack, J.J. Elevated alpha-Fetoprotein in a Neonate with Benign Hemangioendothelioma of the Liver. *Pediatrics* 1987; 80: 596–597.

[21] Sari, N.; Yalcin, B.; Akyuz, C.; Halioglu, M.; Buyukpamukcu M. Infantile Hepatic Hemangioendothelioma with Elevated Serum alpha-Fetoprotein. *Pediatr Hematol Oncol* 2006; 23: 639–647.

[22] Kelli, S. Serum Markers in Tumor Diagnosis and Treatment. In *Paediatric Oncology-Clinical Practice and Controversies*, 3rd ed; Pinkerton, R., Plowan, P.N., Pieters, R., Eds. London, UK: Edward Arnold Publishers, 2004; pp. 169–188.

[23] Van Tornout, J.M.; Buckley, J.D.; Quinn, J.J; Freusner, J.H.; Krailo, M.D.; King, D.R.; Hammond, G.D.; Ortega, J.A. Timing and Magnitude of Decline in alpha-Fetoprotein Levels in Treated Children with Unresectable or Metastatic Hepatoblastoma are Predictors of Outcome: A Report from the Children's Cancer Group. *J Clin Oncol* 1997; 15: 1190–1197.

[24] Lovvorn, H.N. III; Ayers, D.; Zhao, Z.; Hilmes, M.; Prasad, P.; Shinall, M.C., Jr.; Berch, B.; Neblett, W.W., III; O'Neill, J.A., Jr. Defining Hepatoblastoma Responsiveness to Induction Therapy as Measured by Tumor Volume and Serum alpha-Fetoprotein Kinetics. *J Pediatr Surg* 2010; 45: 121–128.

[25] Clericuzio, C.L.; Chen, E.; McNeil, D.E.; O'Connor, T.; Zackai, E.; Medne, L.; Tonlinson, G.; DeBaun, M. Serum alpha Fetoprotein Screening for Hepatoblastoma in Children with Beckwith-Wiedemann Syndrome or Isolated Hemihyperplasia. *J Pedaitr* 2003; 143(2): 270–272.

[26] Ortega, J.A.; Douglass, E.C.; Feusner, J.H.; Reynolds, M.; Quinn, J.J.; Finegold, M.J.; Haas, J.E.; King, D.R.; Liu-Mares, W.; Sensel, M.G.; Krailo, M.D. Randomized Comparison of Cisplatin/Vincristine/Fluoruracil and Cisplatin/continuous Infusion Doxorubicin for Treatment of Pediatric Hepatoblastoma: A Report from the Children's Cancer Group and the Pediatric Oncology Group. *J Clinl Oncol* 2000; 18(14): 2665–2675.

[27] Sayar, D.; Yaniv, I.; Goshen, Y.; Cohen, I.J. Treatment of alpha-Fetoprotein Secreting Hepatoblastoma by Response of Serum alpha-Fetoprotein Levels: A New Concept. *Pediatr Hematol Oncol* 2001; 18: 509–518.

[28] De Ioris, M.; Brugieres, L.; Zimmermann, A.; Keeling,J.; Brock, P.; Maibach, R.; Pritchard, J.; Shafford, L.; Zsiros, J.; Czaudzerna, P.; Perilongo, G. Hepatoblastoma with a Low Serum alpha-Fetoprotein Level at Diagnosis: The SIOPEL Group Experience. *Eur J Cancer* 2008; 44: 545–550.

[29] Nickerson, H.J.; Silberman, T.L.; McDonald, T.P. Hepatoblastoma, Thrombocytosis, and Increased Thrombopoietin. *Cancer* 1980; 45: 315–317.

[30] Shafford, E.A.; Pritchard, J. Extreme Thrombocytosis as a Diagnostic Clue to Hepatoblastoma. *Arch Di. Child* 1993; 69: 171.

[31] Komura, E.; Matsumura, T.; Kato, T.; Tahara, T.; Tsunoda, Y.; Sawada, T. Thrombopoietin in Patients with Hepatoblastoma. *Stem Cells* 1998; 16: 329–333.

[32] Perilongo, G.; Rigon, F.; Murgia, A. Oncologic Causes of Precocious Puberty. *Pediatr Hematol Oncol* 1989; 6: 331–340.

[33] Grunewald, T.G.; von Luettichau, I.; Welsch, U.; Dorr, H.G.; Hopner, F.; Kovacs, K.; Burdach, S.; Rabl, W. First Report of Ectopic ACTH Syndrome and PTHrP-induced

Hypercalcemia Due to a Hepatoblastoma in a Child. *Eur J Endocrinol* 2010; 162: 813–818.

[34] Czauderna, P.; Mackinlay, G.; Perilongo, G.; Brown, J.; Shafford, E.; Aronson, D.; Pritchard, J.; Chapchap, P.; Keeling, J.; Plaschkes J.; Otte, J.B. Hepatocellular Carcinoma in Children: Results of the First Prospective Study of the International Society of Pediatric Oncology Group. *J Clin Oncol* 2002; 12: 2798–2804.

[35] Bellani, F.F.; Massimino, M. Liver Tumors in Childhood: Epidemiology and Clinics. *J Surg Onc* 1993; Suppl 3: 119–121.

[36] Walther, A.; Tiao, G. Approach to Pediatric Hepatocellular Carcinoma. *Clin Liver Dis* 2013; 2: 219–222.

[37] Fukuda, A.; Sakamoto, S.; Kanazawa, H.; Shigeta, T.; Karaki, C.; Hamano, I.; Uchida, H.; Kitagawa, U.; Okuse, C.; Miyazaki, O.; Nosaka, S.; Nakazawa, A.; Kasahara, A. Incidentally Detected Cholangiocarcinoma in an Explanted Liver with Biliary Atresia after Kasai Operation. *Pediatr Transplant* 2013; E: 62–66.

[38] Roth, A. An Unusual Renal Tumor, Associated Nephroblastoma, Nephroblastomatosis, Teratoma, and Cystic Dysplasia with Arterial Hypertension and Secretion of alpha-Fetoprotein. *J Urol (Paris)* 1984; 90: 7–10.

[39] Erol, K.; Vedat, K.; Erkanm D.; Mustafa, G.; Duygu, H.; Avni, A.A. Wilms Tumor Associated with Elevated alpha-Fetoprotein Level. *Pediatr Blood Cancer* 2005; 44: 423–424.

[40] Patriarca, C.; Orazi, A.; Massimino, M.; Luksch, R. A Cystic Partially Differentiated Nephroblastoma Producing alpha-Fetoprotein. *Am J Pediatr Hematol Oncol* 1992; 12: 352–355.

[41] Crocoli, A.; Madafferi, S.; Jenkner, A.; Zaccara, A.; Inserra, A. Elevated Serum alpha-Fetoprotein in Wilms Tumor May Follow the Same Pattern of Other Fetal Neoplasms After Treatment: Evidence from Three Cases. *Pediatr Surg Int* 2008; 24: 499–502.

[42] Dhungel, S.; Cheng, L.J.; Hai, Z.Z. Elevated Serum alpha-Fetoprotein in Wilms' Tumor: A Case Report with Review of Literature. *J Pediatr Surg Case Rep* 2014; 2: 153–155.

[43] Chan, M.H.M.; Shing, M.M.K.; Poon, T.C.W.; Johnson, P.J.; Lam, C.W.K. alpha-Fetoprotein Variants in A Case of Pancreatoblastoma. *Ann Clin Biochem* 2000; 37: 681–685.

[44] Iseki, M.; Suzuki, T.; Koizumi, Y.; Hirose, M.; Laskin, W.B.; Nakazawa, S.; Ohaki, Y. Alpha-Fetoprotein-Producing Pancreatoblastoma. *Cancer* 1986; 57: 1833–1835.

[45] Morohoshi, T.; Sagawa, F.; Mitsuya, T. Pancreatoblastoma with Marked Elevation of Serum alpha-Fetoprotein. *Virchows Archiv A Pathol Anat* 1990; 416: 265–270.

[46] Murray, M.J.; Nicholson, J.C. α-Fetoprotein. *Arch Dis Child Educ Pract Ed* 2011; 96: 141–147.

[47] Murray, M.J.; Halsall, D.J.; Hook, C.E.; Williams, D.M.; Nicholson, J.C.; Coleman, N. Identification of microRNAs rom the miR-371-373 and miR-302 Clusters as Potential Serum Biomarkers of Malignant Germ Cell Tumors. *Am J Clin Pathol* 2011; 135:119–125.

[48] Murray, M.J.; Nicholson, J.C.; Coleman, N. Biology of Childhood Germ Cell Tumour, Focusing on the Significance of microRNAs. *Andrology* 2014.doi: 10.111/andr.277

Section 4

RDTs' in Diagnosis of Drug-Induced Immediate-Type Hypersensitivity

Chapter 4

The Performance of Flowcytometry-Assisted Basophil Activation Tests in the Diagnosis of Drug-Induced Immediate-Type Hypersensitivity Reactions

Cristina Petrişor, Manuela Sfichi, Nadia Gherman,
Mihaela Cociş and Natalia Hagău

Additional information is available at the end of the chapter

http://dx.doi.org/10.5772/64178

Abstract

Background: Flowcytometry-assisted basophil activation tests (BAT) are useful in vitro diagnostic tools for drug-induced immediate-type hypersensitivity.

Objective: The study aimed to perform a medical literature review on the performance of CD63 BAT.

Results: Seven studies for antibiotics, eleven for neuromuscular blocking agents (NMBAs), and 10 for nonsteroidal anti-inflammatory drugs (NSAIDs) were included. The reference standards such as history, skin tests, challenge tests, and/or IgE, along with the concentrations, varied among studies. The thresholds for BAT positivity varied from basophils in the range greater than 4–15%, a net percentage of activated basophils greater than 5% or a stimulation index ranging 1.76–1.85, to the use of more complex composite indexes for NMBAs. For antibiotics and NSAIDs, a stimulation index > 2 was generally chosen. BAT sensitivity for β-lactams was 33–55%, while specificity was 79–93.3%. For NMBAs, BAT sensitivity was 36–92%, while specificity was 93–100%. For NSAIDs, BAT sensitivity was 11.7–61% and specificity was 74–100%.

Discussion: BAT for the diagnosis of drug hypersensitivity has good specificity, but only moderate sensitivity. Despite the shortcomings and the methodological differences in BAT, the potential benefits to avoid challenge tests and increase the allergologic survey sensitivity have led to their widespread use in the clinical practice and warrant their future standardization.

Keywords: Basophils, Drug, Hypersensitivity, Sensitivity, Specificity

1. Introduction

Flowcytometry-assisted basophil activation tests (BAT) are useful functional in vitro diagnostic tools available to confirm drug-induced immediate-type hypersensitivity reactions. In order to confirm previous hypersensitivity reactions caused by drugs and to identify safe alternatives, rapid and reliable diagnostic tests are needed.

Drug-induced immediate-type hypersensitivity reactions include localized skin rashes, pruritus, and urticaria as minor manifestations, while angioedema, bronchospasm, hypotension, and cardiac arrest are the possible severe life-threatening clinical manifestations [1]. Thus, the main characteristics of the retrospective diagnostic tests should be a high sensitivity to identify and confirm the previous clinical reaction in order to avoid further re-exposure and a high specificity, drug hypersensitivity representing a low-prevalence disease.

The retrospective diagnosis is established by performing a comprehensive allergological survey that includes the history, the allergological work-up, and laboratory diagnostic tests. In vivo comprising the skin prick tests, the intradermal tests, and the challenge tests carry the risk of exposing the patient to the potential culprit drug, cannot be performed in patients who reject their performance, and in pregnant women. They remain, however, the main diagnostic tests in the investigation guidelines and the reference tests for the detection of the in vitro tests' performance.

The current guidelines recommend drug-specific IgE antibody dosing as the main in vitro diagnosis [2–4]. However, the performance of such tests varied in previous reports and the accuracy is not 100%. Moreover, serum total IgE influences the results of the assays for β-lactam-specific antibody dosing [5]. For the neuromuscular blocking agents (NMBAs), previous studies reported that healthy controls might have uneventful exposures despite positive-specific IgE for muscle relaxants [6, 7].

In the last two decades, studies have focused on the cellular tests: the histamine release tests and the basophil activation tests, which can confirm IgE- and non-IgE-mediated reactions. Flowcytometry-assisted basophil activation tests are useful in vitro diagnostic tools available to confirm drug-induced immediate-type hypersensitivity reactions. The principle of BAT is to quantify, after the basophils come in contact with the allergen, the upregulation of certain activation markers on the cellular surface by staining with specific fluorescent monoclonal antibodies. The use of BAT allows the rapid confirmation of the previous reaction to the culprit drug (the results can be obtained in less than 3 h), together with the avoidance of another exposure during testing. The performance of BAT for drug hypersensitivity has moderate to low sensitivity, ranging from 33% to 75%, while the reported specificity displayed values >80% [1, 3, 8–11]. However, the studies are not comparable as the inclusion criteria for the study populations, as well as the reference tests varied. Few single-drug studies have been published to investigate the most discriminative threshold to accurately identify patients. The testing methodology and drug concentrations varied from one study to another. No standardized technique currently exists for BAT, but recent advances have improved the performance of this assay [3].

In drug hypersensitivity reactions, extensive research needs have been identified. Among them, one can find the standardization of the test procedures, the development of new diagnostic tools, and the improvement of the already available ones, together with the development of multicenter studies on drug hypersensitivity diagnosis [12].

Despite the shortcomings of the basophil activation tests, their benefit in patients with severe reactions who might avoid challenge tests or the potential to increase the allergologic survey sensitivity have led to their widespread use in the clinical practice and warrant their future standardization.

2. Objectives

In the context of large variability in previous studies on BAT using CD63 as activation marker on the surface of the basophils to quantify the intensity of the immune response that characterizes drug-induced anaphylaxis, the objectives of this review are to underline the methodological differences in previous studies, to identify the optimal drug concentrations to be used in BAT, the optimal incubation conditions, the optimal time frame for testing, and to approximate BAT's performance in terms of sensitivity and specificity.

3. Methods

We performed a scientific literature review on BAT for drug-induced immediate-type hypersensitivity reactions by searching several medical electronic libraries (PubMed, Web of Knowledge, EBSCO, and EMBASE) using keywords such as basophil activation test, drug allergy, drug hypersensitivity, sensitivity, and specificity, in order to identify the published studies on CD63 BAT. In addition, other papers were selected from the references of the previously identified studies. The key elements we searched for included the methodology of BAT, the drug concentrations that were used in BAT, the incubation conditions, the time frame for testing, and BAT's performance in terms of sensitivity and specificity. All studies upon drug-induced immediate-type hypersensitivity reactions were included: antibiotics, nonsteroidal anti-inflammatory drugs (NSAIDs), and NMBAs, as well as reports on miscellaneous rare drug allergies. We excluded review papers, letters to the editors, and editorials.

4. Results

Using the keywords such as basophil activation test, drug allergy, drug hypersensitivity, sensitivity and specificity, we identified over 20 review papers, editorials, and invited commentaries, which we excluded, together with all fundamental in vitro studies on BAT for drugs, in which sensitivity and specificity were not assessed. We included seven papers for antibiotics, eleven studies for NMBAs, and ten studies for NSAID's immediate-type hypersensitivity reactions, all of which evaluated the performance of BAT.

4.1. Antibiotic agents

For antibiotics, we identified seven studies in which BAT sensitivity and specificity were assessed for β-lactams. The reference tests that were considered for comparison varied from history only to the performance of the skin tests and the challenge tests and even to the inclusion of drug-specific IgE dosing (**Table 1**). The optimal threshold for positivity was generally a stimulation index (SI) >2 and a percentage of activated basophils >5%, as identified by the receiver operating characteristic (ROC) curve analysis in several studies [13–15]. It was demonstrated by performing the ROC curve analysis that the SI varies from 1.2 to 3, depending on the tested drug and its concentrations [14]. There was a wide variability concerning the tested drug dilutions. For example, for penicillin G, the tested dilutions were 2 and 0.4 [14–16], 1, 0.1, and 0.01 [17], 3.9 and 0.975 [13], and 2, 0.2, and 0.02 mg/mL [18]. The sensitivity of BAT for β-lactam antibiotics was found to be 33–55%, while the specificity was higher 79–93.3%.

Reference	Threshold for positivity	Se%	Spe%	N	Reference
H, ST	SI > 2, Ba% > 5%, **ROC**	50	93	88	[13]
H, ST, IgEs	SI > 2, Ba% > 5%	49	91	110	[16]
H, ST	CN+6%	33	79	41	[17] **amoxicillin**
H, ST, IgEs	SI > 2, Ba% > 5%, **ROC**	48.3	88.9	262	[14]
H, (ST-)	SI > 2, Ba% > 5%	39.1	93.3	53	[19]
H, ST	SI > 2, Ba% > 5%, **ROC**	55	80	39	[15] **cefuroxime**
H, ST	SI > 1.97, Ba% > 5% - **ROC**	51.4	90.3	68	[18]

H, history; ST, skin tests; IgEs, drug-specific antibodies; SI, stimulation index; Ba%, percentage of activated basophils; ROC, receiver operating characteristic curve analysis used in the study methodology; Se%, sensitivity; Spe%, specificity; N, number of patients and healthy controls included.

Table 1. The performance of BAT for antibiotics.

4.2. NMBAs

For NMBAs, our search retrieved 11 studies reporting the sensitivity and specificity of BAT (**Table 2**). BAT methodology varied between the studies, with one using both CD63 and CD203c as activation markers [20]. BAT sensitivity was 36–92%, depending on the drug to be tested (the highest value was obtained in the study by Ebo et al. for rocuronium [21]), on the severity of the reactions (patients with severe anaphylaxis displaying more often positive results compared to those with cutaneous reactions), as well as on the time frame between the hypersensitivity reaction and testing (higher values were obtained with a time lapse below 3.5 years in the study by Kvedariene et al. [22]). BAT specificity was 93–100%. Studies on BAT for NMBAs initially included patients with immediate-type hypersensitivity to all NMBAs [20, 22–25]. We found that three drug-specific studies (including ours) used ROC curve analysis [21, 26, 27]. The thresholds used for the positivity of BAT varied from activated basophils ranging >4–15%, a net percentage of activated basophils >5% or an SI >1.76–1.85, to the use of more complex composite indexes [28]. There were also differences in the concentrations of NMBAs to be tested, with all research teams using several dilutions starting from the NMBAs available on the market. Optimal concentrations of 500 μg/mL rocuronium and atracurium were identified in drug-specific studies [21, 27].

Reference test	Se%	Spe%	N	Threshold for positivity	Reference
H	64	93	62	↑Ba% > 15%	[23]
H, ST	54	100	60	↑Ba% > 10%	[24]
H	44.44	100	31	↑Ba% > 10%	[20]
H, ST	36-86	93	92	↑Ba% > 15%	[22]
H, ST	92	100	22	Ba% > 4%- **ROC**	[21] **rocuronium**
H, ST, IgEs	68	100	49	Composite index	[28]
H, ST	80	96	104	Net percentage > 4%	[8]
H, ST	68.18	100	56	SI > 1.76, Ba% > 5%- ROC	[25]
H	42.9	90	35	SI > 2	[29]
H, ST	63	100	15	Net percentage > 5%	[13]
H, ST	66.66	100	27	SI > 1.85, Ba% > 5%-**ROC**	[26] **atracurium**

H, history; ST, skin tests; IgEs, drug-specific antibodies; SI, stimulation index; Ba%, percentage of activated basophils; ROC, receiver operating characteristics curve analysis used in the study methodology; Se%, sensitivity; Spe%, specificity; N, total number of patients and healthy controls included.

Table 2. The performance of BAT for NMBAs.

4.3. Nonsteroidal anti-inflammatory drugs (NSAIDs)

We identified 10 studies on aspirin and multiple NSAID-induced hypersensitivity syndrome and three studies on metamizole hypersensitivity (**Table 3**).

History alone or history and the challenge tests represented the reference tests for multiple drug-induced hypersensitivity, starting from the identification of the sensitivity and specificity of BAT [30–34]. In the four studies including ROC curve analysis, an optimal SI >2 and a percentage of activated basophils >5% were found to be most discriminative [30, 32–34]. Using these criteria, the sensitivity of BAT varied widely from 11.7 to 61%, depending on the drug that was tested and the concentrations that were used in the test, while the specificity was 74–100% (**Table 3**).

For metamizole, there were three studies to assess BAT sensitivity and specificity [35–37] (**Table 3**). In the three studies that included ROC curve analysis to identify the optimal cutoff for positivity, SI varied from an SI >5 [35] to an SI >2 [37]. We identified an optimal SI >1.71 from the ROC analysis. Using this lower cutoff, we obtained a sensitivity of 70%, the highest recorded (**Table 3**) [36]. The methodology of BAT differed greatly concerning the drug dilutions that were tested. Gamboa et al. used 5 and 1 mg/mL and Gomez et al. 2.5 and 0.25 mg/mL, while we used lower concentrations such as 25, 2.5, and 0.25 μg/mL [36]. The specificity of BAT for metamizole was 85.71–100%.

Reference test	Se%	Spe%	N	Threshold for positivity	Reference
H, ST, PT	42	100	56	SI > 5 - **ROC**	[35] **metamizole**
H,ST	54.9	85.71	107	SI > 2, Ba% > 5% - **ROC**	[37] **metamizole**
H, ST	70	100	30	SI > 1.71 - **ROC**	[13] **metamizole**
H, PT	15-55	74-100	90	SI > 2, Ba% > 5% - ROC	[30]
H	43	100	72	SI > 5	[31]
H, PT	11.7-41.7	93.3-100	90	SI > 2, Ba% > 5%	[32]
H,PT	76.7	80	45	Ba > 4.58 - ROC	[38]
H	61	91	29	SI > 2, Ba% > 5% - **ROC**	[13]
H	37	90	80	SI > 2, Ba% > 5% - **ROC**	[34]
H,PT	21.7-55.5	51.1-91.1	91	SI > 2, Ba% > 5%	[39]

H, history; ST, skin tests; IgEs, drug-specific antibodies; SI, stimulation index; Ba%, percentage of activated basophils; ROC, receiver operating characteristic curve analysis used in the study methodology; Se%, sensitivity; Spe%, specificity; N, number of patients and healthy controls included.

Table 3. The sensitivity and specificity of BAT for NSAIDs.

5. Discussion

5.1. Epidemiologic characteristics of drug-induced hypersensitivity and allergologic diagnosis

Drug allergy is a significant health problem with serious consequences of diagnostic errors [8, 40]. Most frequently, immediate-type hypersensitivity reactions triggered by drug agents are caused by β-lactam antibiotics and NSAIDs in the general population [41].

Anaphylaxis in the setting of anesthesia is a rare, but potentially lethal, event [42]. NMBAs account for a significant number of intra-anesthetic drug hypersensitivity reactions, followed by antibiotics, hypnotics, analgesics, latex, and chlorhexidine, the latter being frequently overlooked [43–46]. The investigation of adverse reactions to drugs administered in anesthetic conditions and in the perioperative period should be performed in specialized centers and in close collaboration with anesthetists [2, 47].

The diagnosis of an immediate-type hypersensitivity begins with the clinical history and physical examination, confirmed through skin tests and allergen specific IgE measurement [48, 49]. After more than a century of relying on skin testing and 40 years of relying on quantification of specific IgE antibodies in drug allergy diagnosis, clinicians now have access to flow-assisted quantification of activated basophils [50]. To date, BAT is used in more than 50% of the drug allergy centers [51].

5.2. The principle for the basophil activation tests for drugs

Basophils are the rarest granulocytes and represent one of the most enigmatic cells, whose precise biological roles in allergic responses and immune regulation are still unclear [52–55].

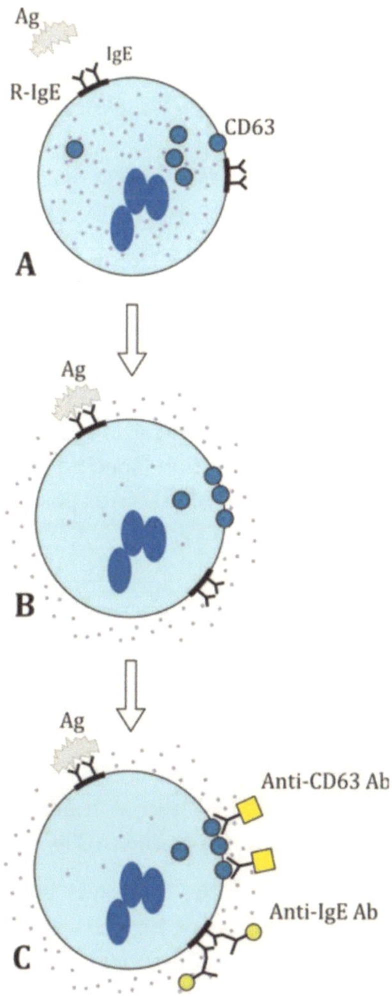

Figure 1. The basophil activation test steps: (A) basophils in contact with the culprit drug in vitro; (B) basophil degranulation after the contact with the allergen, the expression of CD63 activation markers on the cellular membrane; (C) identification of the reactive cells after double staining with monoclonal antibodies. Ag, antigen; IgE-R, the surface receptor for IgE; Ab, antibody. Adapted from [59].

The intensity of the immune response that characterizes anaphylaxis can be detected in vitro when the blood basophils (the key cells in peripheral blood involved in the development of anaphylaxis) are exposed to the culprit drug, the antigen. Thus, BAT represents a functional diagnostic tool [56]. The activation of the basophils involves complex immunological mechanisms, with intracellular changes followed by the release of the mediators in the systemic circulation. CD63 is a transmembrane protein which is anchored in the basophil membrane and is exposed on the cellular surface upon activation [20, 57, 58]. The principle of BAT is to quantify, after the basophils come in contact with the allergen, the upregulation of certain activation markers such as CD63 on the cellular surface by staining with fluorescent, specific monoclonal antibodies (**Figure 1**, adapted from [59]).

CD63 is expressed on the surface of the basophils upon contact with the allergen. CD203c is constitutively expressed on basophils. Both markers have been studied, but most published data have included CD63 flow-assisted BAT [40, 56, 60].

5.3. Flow-assisted basophil activation test: technique

Different protocols and commercial kits are available for BAT [40]. We described the basophil activation test with the quantification of the CD63 activation marker on the surface of the basophils using monoclonal antibodies [61], as follows:

1. Fresh whole blood is needed for the assay and collected into K-EDTA tubes, from a peripheral vein, without using a tourniquet.
2. The assay is performed immediately, without storing blood. We used stimulation buffer as a negative control and anti-FcεRI solution (specific monoclonal antibody for the IgE receptor) and FMLP solution (N-Formyl-Met-Leu) as positive controls. Blood samples are exposed to the culprit drug.
3. Following basophil stimulation with the culprit drug, 20-μL staining reagent and two monoclonal antibodies are added in each tube. We used anti-CCR3-PE (human chemokine receptor coupled with phycoerythrin) and anti-CD63-FITC (a glycoprotein expressed on activated basophils coupled with fluorescein isothiocyanate) as staining reagents.
4. Incubation time is 15 min at 37°C. A prewarmed lysis solution of 2 mL is added to each tube and further incubation lasts for 10 min at room temperature. The samples are centrifuged. Afterwards, the cells are suspended in 300 μL wash buffer.
5. The upregulation of CD63 marker on the basophils is measured. The flowcytometry technique, which implies the detection of forward and side scatter, necessitates the analysis of at least 500 cells in drug allergy diagnosis. The basophils are characterized by low side scattering, and the percentage of CD63-positive cells compared to the total amount of gated basophils is calculated (**Figure 2**, adapted from [61]).
6. The results can be expressed as the percentage of activated basophils, the stimulation index (SI), or as the net percentage of activated basophils. SI is calculated as the percentage of activated basophils after stimulation with the culprit drug divided by the negative control. The net percentage of the activated basophils is calculated by subtracting the negative control from the value obtained with drug stimulation. An additional criterion

http://dx.doi.org/10.5772/64178

necessitates the percentage of activated basophils to be >5% in order to avoid small, unspecific stimulation.

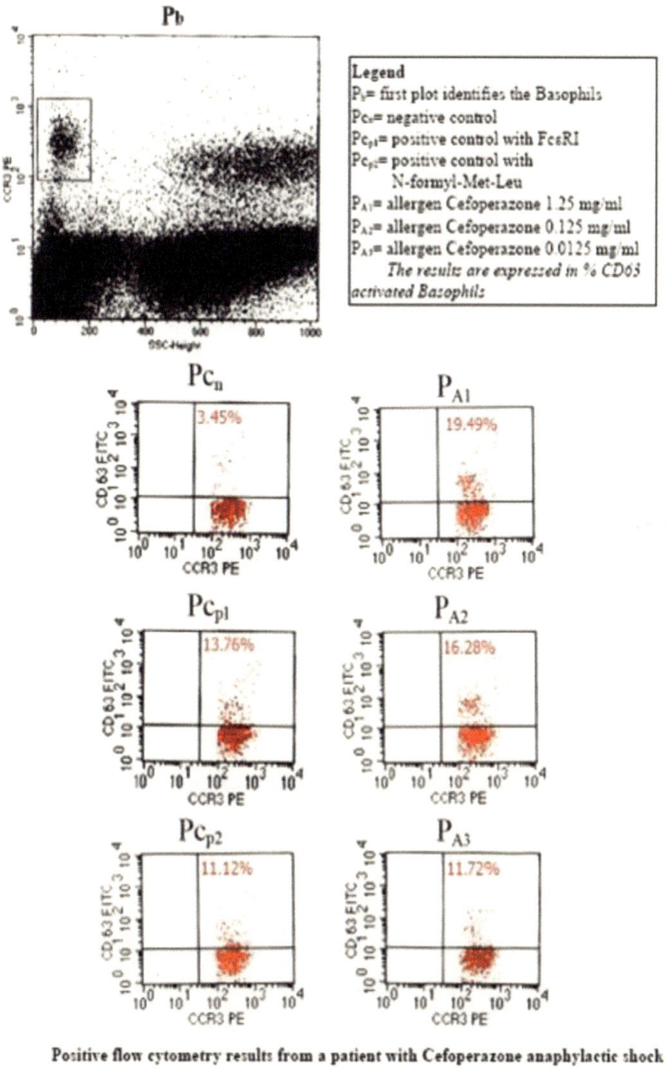

Figure 2. The basophil activation test results in a patient with previous intraanesthetic anaphylactic shock caused by cefoperazone. Adapted from [61].

5.4. Potential benefits and technical challenges in flowcytometry techniques

BAT is a rapid test (results are available within 3 h), and the amount of blood that is required is minimal. BAT reproduces in vitro the immunological hypersensitivity reactions that are induced in vivo when the patient is exposed to the culprit drug. Thus, potentially dangerous re-exposures during the skin tests or the challenge tests are avoided. BAT allows the simultaneous evaluation of several drugs, including therapeutic alternatives and cross-reactive compounds. It can be used in pregnant patients and in those with dermographism, when in vivo tests are contraindicated or the results cannot be interpreted. It is useful for the investigation of clinical reactions that were suspected to be caused by histamine-releasing drugs such as atracurium and morphine, for which the skin tests are false positive due to the local release of histamine. BAT could confirm IgE- and non-IgE-mediated immediate-type hypersensitivity reactions.

The technical challenges of BAT, which restrict its use to specialized centers, are as follows:

- There is no activation marker with 100% specificity for the basophils.
- There is wide interindividual variability regarding the density of IgE receptors on the surface of the cells.
- The minimum number of gated basophils is 200, as this cell population can present variable responses to stimulation.
- The flow analysis is temperature dependent, requires an optimal incubation period (15–20 min), and requires specific buffer solutions and drug concentrations.
- The use of anti-IgE antibodies can stain other cells such as monocytes, eosinophils, and dendritic cells, which present the IgE receptors on their surface.
- Anti-IgE and IL-3, which is used for priming, can activate basophils in high doses.
- The standardization of the techniques is difficult to achieve.

5.5. Current knowledge on the performance of BAT for drug hypersensitivity in view of the STARD criteria

The evaluation of the performance of diagnostic tests, expressed in terms of sensitivity and specificity, can be done using the receiver operating characteristics curves (ROC curves) (**Figure 3**, adapted from [18]) [62]. Using this first method, an optimal threshold is identified, together with the test's sensitivity and specificity [26]. Another method to estimate the diagnostic accuracy would be to calculate sensitivity by dividing number of patients with positive BAT by the total number of investigated patients, while specificity is calculated as the ratio between the number of controls with negative BAT divided by the total number of healthy controls, assuming that the threshold for positivity is well-known and accepted. Both methods have been used in the diagnosis of immediate-type hypersensitivity reactions triggered by drugs. The latter method has been used for basophil activation test, using the cutoff identified for other allergens and antibiotics in the studies on other drugs, which rarely cause drug hypersensitivity, such as the NMBAs [8, 25]. The diagnostic accuracy of the tests could be improved by applying specific cutoffs. For drug allergy diagnosis, it is essential that an adequate number of allergic patients and healthy controls are included in the ROC analysis to determine the most discriminative thresholds for positivity [40, 42].

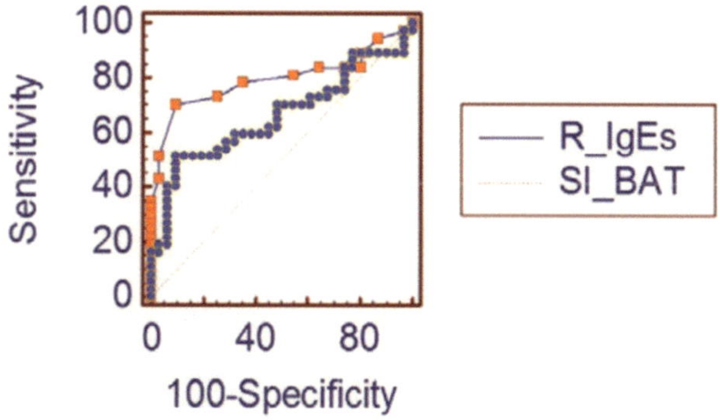

Figure 3. Receiver operating characteristics (ROC) curves for two in vitro techniques: radioimmunoassay (R) and flow-cytometry (BAT) for β-lactam antibiotic hypersensitivity. Adapted from [18].

The significance of the methodology by which we evaluate BAT performance is remarkable:

- The diagnostic tests for drug-induced immediate-type hypersensitivity reactions need a high sensitivity. A low sensitivity would mean a high number of false-negative results, and consequently the patients could subsequently be at risk upon re-exposure to the culprit drug. False-negative diagnosis can put these patients at risk for severe allergic reactions [17].
- As drug hypersensitivity is a low-prevalence disease, the specificity has to be high as well. A high specificity rarely generates false-positive results and guarantees that a positive result has clinical significance. False-positive results would be disadvantageous as they would result in drug avoidance.

5.6. Allergological survey for the retrospective diagnosis of drug-induced immediate-type hypersensitivity reactions: the reference tests

The retrospective diagnosis of immediate-type hypersensitivity reactions caused by drug agents is established after the performance of a complex allergological survey that includes the history, the allergologic tests, and drug-specific IgE dosing [2].

The history is not always reliable and the differential diagnosis is complex, especially for intra-anesthetic hypersensitivity reactions, when several drugs are administered simultaneously. Skin testing is the most widely used method to determine sensitization [2]. The skin tests have not been evaluated regarding their diagnostic accuracy and need to be performed in an optimal time frame after the reaction [42]. Testing within 4–6 weeks might give false-negative results, as well as testing after several years. The sensitivity and specificity of skin testing can be variable [2, 20]. Thus, the optimal time frame for in vivo studies would be 6 weeks to 6 months after the clinical reaction. Moreover, several categories of patients including pregnant women cannot be skin tested due to the severity of the reaction (patients with previous severe anaphylaxis might not even give consent), as in vivo studies always carry the risk of re-exposure to the culprit drug. The challenge tests cannot be recommended for daily routine, as they are difficult to perform, the standardization is difficult, and they carry the risk of a potentially dangerous re-exposure. Their use is hampered by ethical and practical limitations [40].

The evaluation of the serum tryptase concentration can be carried out in the first few hours following the clinical reaction. While an immediate-type hypersensitivity reaction can be confirmed when the clinical signs are highly suggestive, there are some issues regarding the interpretation of serum tryptase measurement: there is no definitive agreement upon the cutoff value, there can be false-positive results in mastocytosis or severe hypoxemia, as well as false negative when there is sudden cardiac arrest with no or limited cardiac output and blood flow to bring tryptase from the peripheral tissues in the central circulating blood volume [63, 64].

The detection of IgE-type drug-specific antibodies is currently recommended by the clinical guidelines, even though their absolute value is not 100%. They are the most widely used in vitro tests to confirm drug hypersensitivity retrospectively. For β-lactam antibiotics, the results of the tests are altered by the value of the total serum IgE [5], while for NMBAs, specific IgE antibodies were identified in the serum of normal healthy controls, with no clinical reaction upon exposure [6, 40, 65].

None of the available diagnostic methods demonstrates absolute accuracy and the lack of a perfect gold standard test is one of the major problems in drug allergy diagnosis. Therefore, it is difficult to investigate the performance of BAT [8, 27, 42].

Due to the limitations of these diagnostic methods, the performance of cellular functional studies has been introduced in the last two decades. Over 50% of the drug allergy centers use the basophil activation tests in the diagnostic algorithms [51].

5.7. BAT for antibiotics hypersensitivity

Characteristic of antibiotics, loss of sensitivity naturally occurs over time. First, several years after a clinical reactions, the results of the skin tests may be negative and the patient might need to undergo challenge tests. Second, the in vitro diagnosis is challenging as the determination of specific IgE antibodies is only available for a limited number of antibiotics and the immunoassays do not show an absolute accuracy [15, 40].

β-Lactam antibiotics are the drugs that most frequently produce immediate-type hypersensitivity reactions [13, 17]. This explains the fact that the studies on BAT sensitivity and specificity for β-lactam antibiotics include a large number of patients and do not show extensive heterogeneity, as for NMBAs. For example, most of the studies, except one, used an optimal SI >2 and Ba% >5% as positivity cutoffs, as identified by the performance of the ROC curve analysis (**Table 1**). The first multicenter European study that addressed in vitro drug allergy diagnosis using BAT was performed for β-lactams [14].

BAT sensitivity is close to that of IgE immunoassays, but the use of both diagnostic tests improves sensitivity [14, 16]. BAT and IgE are complementary and allow the increase of the allergologic survey sensitivity when decision algorithms are used. The number of patients with positive history and negative diagnostic tests is reduced when several diagnostic methods are used [14, 18]. Although BAT has moderate sensitivity, it could allow the avoidance of challenge tests in patients with negative skin tests and positive BAT results [40]. The use of BAT in patients with negative skin tests might allow the avoidance of challenge tests in patients with hypersensitivity, but whose skin sensitivity has diminished in time.

Few reports have also been published on allergies to antibiotics, other than β-lactams, for instance, quinolones [66, 67]. In these cases, BAT was performed for the retrospective confirmation of a clinical reaction using the cutoffs identified for the β-lactams.

5.8. BAT for NMBAs hypersensitivity

Muscle relaxants are the main cause of anaphylaxis during anesthesia [63, 68]. The diagnosis of NMBA allergy remains particularly difficult: during anesthesia, several drugs are administered in a short period of time; the histamine-releasing NMBAs might show false-positive skin tests results if the testing concentrations are higher than recommended, while it is difficult to perform challenge tests due to ethical and methodological issues [2, 40]. Even though the skin tests have no absolute predictive values, they remain the reference standard for the diagnosis in this context [24]. In previous studies, inclusion criteria varied from history alone to history and skin test results and even positive IgEs (**Table 2**). This inclusion variability could be in part responsible for the differences in the reported BAT sensitivity and specificity. NMBA allergy is a low-prevalence disease, making the recruitment of well-defined patients difficult. Thus, in the first studies, patients with hypersensitivity reactions caused by NMBAs were included in the analysis, and the assessment of BAT performance was done for this class of drugs using arbitrarily defined cutoffs [20, 22–24]. Only in recent years, few drug-specific studies used the ROC curve analysis, which included a limited number of patients and identified optimal thresholds for positivity [21, 26, 27]. The manufacturers recommend the use of an SI >2 as the cutoff for positivity, by extrapolating from the antibiotic and NSAID studies on drug hypersensitivity, which included a larger number of patients. However, it is difficult to justify the use of a single cutoff for all drugs, as the stimulation conditions might differ considerably from NMBA to NMBA [21]. The methodology and optimal decision thresholds for BAT vary considerably from one study to another [26]. Among all the drugs, BAT for NMBAs displays the highest degree of variability regarding the inclusion criteria and positivity thresholds.

We have identified an optimal SI >1.76 for NMBAs as a class and an optimal SI >1.85 for atracurium [25, 26]. By lowering the threshold for positivity, the sensitivity of the assay might be increased. As anaphylaxis from NMBAs can be a threat to the patients' life, it is critical to establish a sensitive cutoff [21]. The time frame for testing was also important; higher sensitivities were achieved when the tests were performed 6 weeks to 3.5 years after the clinical reaction and when the reaction was severe [22].

Moreover, the concentrations for the tested NMBAs varied considerably in the studies, and it seems that each drug might have different optimal concentrations [40].

There was no perfect correlation between the clinical assessment of the disease and the biological tests such as BAT and IgE, suggesting that they investigate potentially different immunological mechanisms and the need to be used complementary [24]. BAT can add to the diagnosis of NMBA allergy especially when the skin test results are negative and inconclusive [40].

BAT confirms previous reactions caused by drug agents and might allow the clinician chose a safe alternative for future anesthesia [27, 40].

5.9. BAT for NSAIDs hypersensitivity

NSAIDs are the second group of drugs responsible for anaphylaxis [34, 69]. The evaluation of BAT performance for the diagnosis of NSAID hypersensitivity is even more complex due to the clinical spectrum of the reactions. Several types of hypersensitivity reactions have been defined. First, an immediate-type hypersensitivity reaction is related to COX-1 inhibition, which is induced by multiple NSAIDs and displays cross-reactivity in the same patient for several drugs from this class. Second, single-drug-induced immediate-type hypersensitivity reaction was defined, which is mediated by IgE [69].

For NSAIDs, the oral challenge tests are the reference standards for drug allergy diagnosis and there are no commercialized in vitro assays to detect specific IgE, which is not the mechanism in multiple drug hypersensitivity [33]. Thus, reliable in vitro tools are required to confirm this type of drug-induced hypersensitivity. BAT is not the first test that is recommended in the allergological workup for NSAID hypersensitivity, but it can be used in addition to other diagnostic methods, even though heterogenous results have been obtained regarding its performance for this class of drugs [37].

Whether BAT is useful for multiple NSAID-induced hypersensitivity syndrome has been debated in previous studies, as the sensitivity of the test was generally low and varied widely, in part due to different methodologies and drug concentrations that were used. Thus, the reliability of NSAID-induced basophil activation determined by flowcytometry has been questioned. Clinically validated and standardized studies, that include a large number of patients, are still awaited for BAT in this field of multiple NSAID-induced hypersensitivity diagnosis and further development is required to increase the sensitivity of the test [33, 39]. Up to date, no universal in vitro test, which would be applicable to the diagnosis of all types of NSAID hypersensitivity, can be recommended [69].

The three studies on metamizole hypersensitivity diagnosis are not comparable as the drug dilutions used in BAT differed, as well as the threshold for positivity which was obtained by ROC analysis. We have shown that by lowering the threshold and using lower concentrations of metamizole, the sensitivity of the test can be improved, without diminishing the specificity [36]. As drug anaphylaxis can be severe, any improvements in BAT methodology, which have a positive impact on the sensitivity of the test, deserve attention.

5.10. BAT for miscellaneous drugs and rare drug allergies

Several case reports on BAT confirm immediate-type hypersensitivity reactions caused by biological drugs, radiocontrast media, and methylprednisolone [70–73]. In these cases, the extremely low incidence of the disease will not allow the identification of optimal incubation conditions, concentrations, and cutoffs, to estimate the performance of BAT.

6. Conclusions

The current limitations for the use of basophil activation tests in the retrospective diagnosis of immediate-type hypersensitivity reactions caused by drugs arise from the low prevalence of the disease, limiting the number of patients in the clinical studies, and from the lack of a gold standard test with absolute accuracy, together with the use of surrogate reference tests in the studies. There was a wide variability in the methodology of BAT for drugs concerning the concentrations used in the test and the optimal thresholds for positivity chosen and how these were identified. BAT for drug hypersensitivity has good specificity, but only moderate sensitivity, which needs to be improved in future. BAT could be improved using other activation markers, by new gating strategies to capture basophils and possibly by building a consensus guideline for its standardization [74].

Despite the shortcomings of the currently available BAT techniques and the methodological differences, the benefits of using rapid cellular tests in patients with severe reactions, thus avoiding challenge tests or the potential to increase the allergologic survey sensitivity by the combined use of several in vitro tests, have led to their widespread use in clinical practice and warrant their future standardization. Larger study populations from multicenter studies and a standardized methodological approach are needed to better assess the performance of BAT in terms of sensitivity and specificity for drug-induced immediate-type hypersensitivity reactions.

7. Executive summary

1. The use of BAT allows the rapid confirmation of the previous reaction to the culprit drug in patients with drug hypersensitivity.
2. The main characteristics of the retrospective diagnostic tests for drug hypersensitivity should be high sensitivity to identify and confirm the previous clinical reaction in order to avoid further re-exposure and high specificity as a guarantee that a positive result has clinical significance.
3. None of the available diagnostic methods demonstrates absolute accuracy, and the lack of a perfect gold standard test is one of the major problems in drug allergy diagnosis. In previous studies, inclusion criteria varied from history alone to history and skin test results, and even positive IgEs.
4. The testing methodology and drug concentrations varied from one study to another.
5. Few drug-specific studies used the ROC curve analysis for identifying the optimal threshold for positivity and these included a limited number of patients due to the low prevalence of the disease.
6. Due to methodological differences, previous studies are not comparable.
7. Overall, BAT for drug hypersensitivity has good specificity, but only moderate sensitivity.

8. BAT sensitivity needs to be improved in the future, possibly using new gating strategies to capture the reactive basophils, by adding other activation markers, and by achieving BAT standardization after the performance of multicenter studies that include larger number of patients.

Acknowledgements

Funding was received from "Iuliu Hatieganu" University of Medicine and Pharmacy Cluj-Napoca, internal grant no. 4945/10/08.03.2016.

Author details

Cristina Petrişor[1,2*], Manuela Sfichi[3], Nadia Gherman[2,4], Mihaela Cociş[1] and Natalia Hagău[1,2]

*Address all correspondence to: petrisor.cristina@umfcluj.ro

1 2nd Department of Anaesthesia and Intensive Care, "Iuliu Haţieganu" University of Medicine and Pharmacy Cluj-Napoca, Cluj-Napoca, Romania

2 Clinical Emergency County Hospital of Cluj, Cluj-Napoca, Romania

3 Department of Clinical Immunology, The Clinical Emergency County Hospital Cluj, Cluj-Napoca, Romania

4 Department of Allergology and Immunology, "Iuliu Haţieganu" University of Medicine and Pharmacy Cluj-Napoca, Cluj-Napoca, Romania

References

[1] Rive C, Bourke J, Phillips E. Testing for drug hypersensitivity syndromes. Clin Biochem Rev. 2013; 34:15–38.

[2] Brockow K, Garvey LH, Aberer W, Atanaskovic-Markovic M, Barbaud A, Bilo MB, et al. Skin test concentrations for systemically administered drugs—an ENDA/EAACI Drug Allergy Group position paper. Allergy. 2013;68:702–712.

[3] McGowan E, Saini S. Update on the performance and application of basophil activation tests. Curr Allergy Asthma Rep. 2013;13:101–109.

[4] Romano A, Torres M, Castells M, et al. Diagnosis and management of drug hypersensitivity reactions. J Allergy Clin Immunol. 2011; 127(3):S67–S73.

[5] Petrişor C, Sfichi M, Gherman N, Bologa R, Hagău N. Elevated total serum IgE alter the diagnostic performance of radio-immune assays for β-lactam specific antibody dosing. Clin Lab. 2015;61:149–154.

[6] Petrişor C, Brezoski E, Gherman-Ionică N, Sfichi M, Hagău N. In vitro tests versus skin tests and a positive history of neuromuscular blocking agents-induced immediate-type hypersensitivity reactions. J Rom Anest Terap Int. 2014;21(1):13–18.

[7] Leysen J, Bridts C, De Clerk LS, Vercauteren M, Lambert J, Weyler J. Allergy to rocuronium: from clinical suspicion to correct diagnosis. Allergy. 2011; 66:1014–1019.

[8] Leysen J, Sabato V, Verweij M, De Knop K, Bridts C, De Clerk L. The basophil activation test in the diagnosis of immediate drug hypersensitivity. Expert Rev Clin Immunol. 2011;7(3):349–355.

[9] Mayorga C, Sanz ML, Gamboa PM. *In vitro* diagnosis of immediate allergic reactions to drugs: an update. J Investig Allergol Clin Immunol. 2010;20(2):103–109.

[10] Hausmann OV, Gentinetta T, Bridts CH, Ebo DG. The basophil activation test in immediate-type drug allergy. Immunol Allergy Clin N Am. 2009; 29: 555–566.

[11] Song WJ, Chang YS. Recent applications of basophil activation tests in the diagnosis of drug hypersensitivity. Asia Pac Allergy. 2013;3:266–280.

[12] Papadopoulos N, Agache I, Bavbek S, Bilo P, Braido F, Cardona V. Research needs in allergy: an EAACI position papaer, in collaboration with EFA. Clin Transl Allergy. 2012;2:21.

[13] Sanz ML, Gamboa PM, Antepara I, Uasuf C, Vila L, Garcia-Aviles C. Flow cytometric basophil activation test by detection of CD63 expression in patients with immediate-type reactions to betalactam antibiotics. Clin Exp Allergy. 2002;32: 277–286.

[14] De Weck AL, Sanz ML, Gamboa PM, Aberer W, Sturm G, Bilo MB, and members of ENDA (European Network for Drug Allergy). Diagnosis of immediate-type ß-lactam allergy in vitro by flow-cytometric basophil activation test and sulfidoleukotriene production: a multicenter study. J Investig Allergol Clin Immunol. 2009; 19: 91–109.

[15] Eberlein B, Suarez L, Darsow U, Rueff F, Behrendt H, Ring J. A new basophil activation test using CD63 and CCR3 in allergy to antibiotics. Clin Exp Allergy. 2010; 40 (3): 411–418.

[16] Torres MJ, Padial A, Mayorga C. The diagnostic interpretation of basophil activation test in immediate allergic reactions to betalactams. Clin Exp Allergy. 2004;34:1768–1775.

[17] Abuaf N, Rostane H, Rajoely B, Gaouarw H, Autegardenw JE, Leynadierw F. Comparison of two basophil activation markers CD63 and CD203c in the diagnosis of amoxicillin allergy. Clin Exp Allergy. 2008;38: 921–928.

[18] Petrișor C, Gherman-Ionică N, Bologa R, Sfichi M, Hagău N. Basophil activation test versus radio-immunoassay in the diagnosis of β-lactam immediate-type hypersensitivity reactions. Rom Rev Lab Med. 2013; 21(4):415–422.

[19] Gamboa PM, Garcia-Aviles MC, Urrutia I, Antepara I, Esparza, Sanz ML. Basophil activation and sulfidoleukotriene production in patients with immediate allergy to betalactam antibiotics and negative skin tests. J Invest Allergol Clin Immunol. 2004; 14: 278–283.

[20] Sudheer PS, Hall JE, Read GF, Rowbottom AW, Williams PE. Flow cytometric investigation of peri-anaesthetic anaphylaxis using CD63 and CD203c. Anaesthesia. 2005; 60: 251–256.

[21] Ebo DG, Bridts CH, Hagendorens MM, Mertens CH, De Clerck LS, W. J. Stevens WJ. Flow-assisted diagnostic management of anaphylaxis from rocuronium bromide. Allergy. 2006;61: 935–939.

[22] Kvedariene V, Kamey S, Ryckwaert Y, et al. Diagnosis of neuromuscular blocking agent hypersensitivity reactions using cytofluorimetric analysis of basophils. Allergy. 2006; 61: 311–315.

[23] Abuaf N, Rajoely B, Ghazouani E. Validation of a flow cytometric assay detecting *in vitro* basophil activation for the diagnosis of muscle relaxant allergy. J Allergy Clin Immunol. 1999;104:411–418.

[24] Monneret G, Benoit Y, Debard AL. Monitoring of basophil activation using CD63 and CCR3 in allergy to muscle relaxant drugs. Clin Immunol. 2002;102(2):192–199.

[25] Hagau N, Gherman-Ionica N, Sfichi M, Petrișor C. Threshold for basophil activation test positivity in neuromuscular blocking agent hypersensitivity reactions. Allergy Asthma Clin Immunol. 2013;9:42.

[26] Petrișor C, Gherman N, Sfichi M, Cociș M, Hagău N. Immediate-type hypersensitivity to atracurium: use of the stimulation index as the optimal positivity threshold for the flow-assisted basophil activation test. J Investig Allergol Clin Immunol. 2015;25(5): 372–373.

[27] Uyttebroek AP, Sabato V, Leysen J, Bridts CH, De Clerk LS, Ebo DG. Flowcytometric diagnosis of atracurium-induced anphylaxis. Allergy. 2014;69:1324–1332.

[28] Sainte-Laudy J, Boumediene A, Touraine F, Orsel I, Cogne M. Anaphylaxis of IgE down regulation induced by basophil activation. Application to the diagnosis of muscle relaxant allergic hypersensitivity by flow cytometry. Inflamm Res. 2006;55:S21–22.

[29] Xin X, Yi Z, Lijiao X, Jia Y, Jianqing G, Zixi W, Yuguang H, Jing Z. Investigation of drugs responsible for perioperative anaphylactic reactions using cellular allergen stimulation test. Chin Med J. 2014;127(21):3738–3743.

[30] Gamboa P, Sanz ML, Caballero MR. The flow cytometric determination of basophil activation induced by aspirin and other non-steroidal anti-inflammatory drugs

(NSAIDS) is useful for *in vitro* diagnosis of the NSAIDS hypersensitivity syndrome. Clin Exp Allergy. 2004; 34: 1448–1457.

[31] Rodriguez-Trabado A, Camara-Mijon C, Ramos-Cantarino A. Basophil activation test for the *in vitro* diagnosis of nonsteroidal anti-inflammatory drug hypersensitivity. Allergy Asthma Proc. 2008;29(3):241–249.

[32] Sanz ML, Gamboa P, De Weck AL. A new combined test with flowcytometric basophil activation and determination of sulfidoleukotrienes is useful for in vitro diagnosis of hypersensitivity to aspirin and other nonsteroidal anti-inflammatory drugs. Int Arch Allery Immunol. 2005; 136:58–72.

[33] Kim M, Joo Cho Y. Flow cytometry-assisted basophil activatrion test as a safe diagnostic tool for aspirin/NSAID hypersensitivity. Allergy Asthma Immunol Res. 2012;4(3): 137–142.

[34] Abuaf N, Rostane H, Barbara J. Comparison of CD63 upregulation induced by NSAIDs on basophils and monocytes in patients with NSAID hypersensitivity. J Allergy. 2012;580873.

[35] Gamboa PM, Sanz ML, Caballero MR, Antepara I, Urrutia I, Jauregui I. Use of CD63 expression as a marker of *in vitro* basophil activation and leukotriene determination in dipyrone allergic patients. Allergy. 2003;58: 312–317.

[36] Hagău N, Longrois D, Petrişor C. Threshold for positivity and optimal dipyrone concentration in flow-assisted basophil activation test. Allergy Asthma Immunol Res. 2013;5(6):383–388.

[37] Gómez E, Blanca-Lopez N, Torres MJ, Requena G, Rondon C, Canto G. Immunoglobulin E-mediated immediate allergic reactions to dipyrone: value of basophil activation test in the identification of patients. Clin Exp Allergy. 2009;39:1217–1224.

[38] Wismol P, Putivoranat P, Buranapraditkun S, Pinnobphun S, Ruxrungtham K, Klaewsongkram J. The values of nasal provocation test and basophil activation test in the different patterns of ASA/NSAID hypersensitivity. Allergol Immunopathol. 2011; DOI: 10.1016/j.aller.2010.12.011.

[39] Ariza A, Fernandez T, Dona I. Basophil activation after nonsteroidal anti-inflammatory drug stimulation in patients with immediate hypersensitivity reactions to these drugs. Cytometry (Part A). 2014;85A:400–407.

[40] Ebo DG, Leysen J, Mayorga C. The *in vitro* diagnosis of drug allergy: status and perspectives. Allergy. 2011;66:1275–1286.

[41] Dona I, Blanca-Lopez N, Torres M. Drug hypersensitivity reactions: response patterns, drug involved, and temporal variations in a large series of patients. J Investig Allergol Clin Immunol. 2012;22(5):363–371.

[42] Bleasel K, Donnan G, Unglik G. General anesthetic allergy testing. Curr Allergy Asthma Rep. 2009;9:50–56.

[43] Garvey IH. Practical aspects of perioperative anaphylaxis. Trend Anaesth Crit Care. 2013; 3:320–325.

[44] Gonzales-Estrada A, Pien L, Zell K. Antibiotics are an important cause identifiable cause of perioperative anaphylaxis in the United States. J Allergy Clin Immunol Pract. 2015;3(1):101–105.

[45] Gurrieri C, Weingarten T, Martin D. Allergic reactions during anesthesia at a large United States referral center. Anesth Analg. 2011;113(5):1202–1212.

[46] Mertes P, Alla F, Trechit P. Anaphylaxis during anesthesia in France: an 8-year national survey. J Allergy Clin Immunol. 2011;128(2):366–373.

[47] Guyer A, Staff R, Conroy M. Comprehensive allergy evaluation is useful in the subsequent care of patients with drug hypersensitivity reactions during anesthesia. J Allergy Clin Immunol Pract. 2015; 3(1):94–100.

[48] HE S, Zhang H, Zeng X, Chen D, Yang P. Mast cells and basophils are essential for allergies: mechanism of allergic inflammation and a proposed procedure for diagnosis. Acta Pharmacol Sin. 2013;34:1270–1283.

[49] Mertes PM, Malinovsky JM, Jouffroy L. Reducing the risk of anaphylaxis during anesthesia: 2011 updated guidelines for clinical practice. J Investig Allergol Clin Immunol. 2011;21(6):442–453.

[50] Ebo D, Hagendorens M, Bridts C, Stevens W. *In vitro* diagnosis of IgE-mediated allergy: breakthroughs in the last decade. Expert Rev Clin Immunol. 2012;8(1):9–11.

[51] Thong B, Mirakian R, Castells M, Pichler W, Romano A, Bonnadonna P. A World Allergy Organization international survey on diagnostic procedures and therapies in drug allergy/hypersensitivity. WAO J. 2011;4:257–270.

[52] Gibbs BF, Nilsson GP. Basophils unlimited. Allergy. 2013;68:553–554.

[53] Chirumbolo S. State-of-the-art review about basophil research in immunology and allergy: is the time right to treat these cells with the respect they deserve? Blood Transf. 2012;10:148–164.

[54] Saito H, Ishizaka T, Ishizaka K. Mast cells and IgE: from history to today. Allergol Int. 2013;62:3–12.

[55] Siracusa M, Kim B, Spergel J, Artis D. Basophils and allergic inflammation. J Allergy Clin Immunol. 2013; 132:789–801.

[56] Mobs C, Pfuntzer W. Cellular *in vitro* diagnostics of adverse drug reactions. Allergo J Int. 2014:23:164–171.

[57] Hoffman HJ, Santos AF, Mayorga C. The clinical utility of basophil activation testing in diagnosis and monitoring of allergic disease. Allergy. 2015;70:1393–1405.

[58] Steiner M, Harrer A, Lang R. Basophil activation test for investigation of IgE-mediated mechanisms in drug hypersensitivity. J Vis Exp. 2011;55:e3263.

[59] Petrişor C. Flow cytometry-based improvement for the diagnosis of drug-induced hypersensitivity reactions in the surgical patients. PhD thesis. Cluj-Napoca, Romania: "Iuliu Haţieganu" University of Medicine and Pharmacy; 2014.

[60] MacGlashan D. Basophil activation testing. J Allergy Clin Immunol. 2013;132(4):777–787.

[61] Hagău N, Sfichi M, Bologa R, Cocu S, Indrei C, Alb I, Bene L. Basophil activation test using flow cytometry in the diagnosis of antibiotic allergy. Rom Rev Lab Med. 2010;18:41–47.

[62] Bossuyt PM, Reitsma JB, Bruns DE, Gatsonis CA, Glasziou PP, Irwig L, For the STARD Group. STARD 2015: an updated list of essential items for reporting diagnostic accuracy studies. BMJ. 2015;351:h5527.

[63] Laroche D, Gomis P, Gallimidi E. Diagnostic value of histamine and tryptase concentrations in severe anaphylaxis with shock and cardiac arrest during anesthesia. Anestesiology. 2014;121(2):272–279.

[64] Sheldon J, Philips B. Laboratory investigation of anaphylaxis: not as easy as it seems. Anaesthesia. 2015;70(1):1–5.

[65] Leysen J, Uyttebroek A, Sabato V. Predictive value of allergy tests for neuromuscular blocking agents: tackling an unmet need. Clin Exp Allergy. 2014;44(8):1069–1075.

[66] Aranda A, Mayorga C, Ariza A, et al. *In vitro* evaluation of IgE-mediated hypersensitivity reactions to quinolones. Allergy. 2011;66:247–254.

[67] Ben Said B, Berard F, Bienvenu J. Usefulness of basophil activation test for the diagnosis of IgE-mediated allergy to quinolones. Allergy. 2010;65:534–535.

[68] Aalberse R, Kleine Budde I, Mulder M. Differentiating the cellular and humoral components of neuromuscular blocking agent-induced anaphylacitc reactions in patients undergoing anaesthesia. Br J Anaesth. 2011; 106(5):665–674.

[69] Kowalski ML, Makowska JS, Blanca M. Hypersensitivity to nonsteroidal anti-inflammatory drugs (NSAIDs)—classification, diagnosis and management: review of the EAACI/ENDA and GA2LEN/HANNA. Allergy. 2011; 66: 818–829.

[70] Aranda A, Mayorga C, Ariza A. IgE-mediated hypersensitivity reactions to methylprednisolone. Allergy. 2010;65:1376–1380.

[71] Ben Said B, Leray V, Nicolas A. Methylprednisolone-induced anaphylaxis: diagnosis by skin test and basophil activation test. Allergy. 2010;65:531–536.

[72] Salas M, Gomez F, Fernandez T. Diagnosis of immediate hypersensitivity reactions to radiocontrast media. Allergy. 2013;68:1203–1206.

[73] Corominas M, Gastamiza G, Lobera T. Hypersensitivity reactions to biological drugs. J Investig Allergol Clin Immunol. 2014;24(4):212–225.

[74] Chirumbolo S. Monitoring of CD63% in basophil activation test and suggested new parameters for allergy diagnosis. Inflamm Res. 2012;61:171–176.

Section 5

Novel Rapid Diagnostic Tests: Nano/Microfluidic Technologies and Fusion with DNA Technologies

Chapter 5

Rapid Diagnosis by Microfluidic Techniques

Xiran Jiang, Wenwen Jing, Lulu Zheng,
Wang Zhao and Guodong Sui

Additional information is available at the end of the chapter

http://dx.doi.org/10.5772/63905

Abstract

Pathogenic bacteria in an aqueous or airborne environments usually cause infectious diseases in hospital or among the general public. One critical step in the successful treatment of the pathogen-caused infections is rapid diagnosis by identifying the causative microorganisms, which helps to provide early warning of the diseases. However, current standard identification based on cell culture and traditional molecular biotechniques often depends on costly or time-consuming detection methods and equipments, which are not suitable for point-of-care tests. Microfluidic-based technique has recently drawn lots of attention, due to the advantage that it has the potential of providing a faster, more sensitive, and higher-throughput identification of causative pathogens in an automatic manner by integrating micropumps and valves to control the liquid accurately inside the chips. In this chapter, microfluidic techniques for serodiagnosis of amebiasis, allergy, and rapid analysis of airborne bacteria are described. The microfluidic chips that integrate microcolumns, protein microarray, or a staggered herringbone mixer structure with sample to answer capability have been introduced and shown to be powerful in rapid diagnosis especially in medical fields.

Keywords: microfluidics, serodiagnosis, pathogen analysis, airborne bacteria, cerebrospinal fluid

1. Introduction

For the past decade, many traditional techniques and methods of bioanalysis and diagnosis have reached the technical bottleneck. While researchers have believed the microfluidic technology is becoming a promising alternative to traditional biological techniques as it allows the operating process to complete in a small chip. Since micrometer channels can be fabricated inside a microfluidic chip with simple operating procedures, fluids, reagents, and biological samples can be controlled accurately inside the chip to perform precise analysis and diagnosis. The smaller size and easy fabrication make the microfluidic devices to have many advantages such as portability, lower sample and reagent consumption and cost, less waste, rapid mass and heat transfer, and parallel analysis abilities. Besides, the increase of automation of the operations inside the chips helps to facilitate very accurate reactions that were usually very hard to be run by traditional methods. Considering the above-mentioned advantages, the microfluidic technique has great potential application in rapid diagnostics and point-of-care detections. Furthermore, combination of microfluidics with some traditional biological techniques will offer insights toward applications in biological and medical fields.

2. Microfluidics for rapid serodiagnosis of amebiasis

Entamoeba histolytica is the causative agent of amebiasis, the clinical significance of which has been demonstrated around the world. Thus, a early diagnosis technique that is capable of rapid analysis of *Entamoeba histolytica* is urgent for the disease control and public health concerns.

A microbead-based immune analysis technique was developed by our group using an integrated microfluidic device and recombinant protein (C-Igl) prepared from an *E. coli* strain containing Gal-lectin of *Entamoeba histolytica* [1]. The novel microfluidic technique greatly reduced the processing time (<20 min compared to a couple of hours if using traditional methods and could have potential application on point-of-care diagnosis of amebiasis). Further, the chip is capable of four parallel analyses at one time, which is very promising for high-throughput analysis. Moreover, it is worth mentioning that only 20 μl of the clinical sample was required for each single assay. The low consumption of both samples and reagents makes the technique suitable for widely applications.

The microfluidic chip structure was presented in **Figure 1**, consisting a bottom control layer and a upper fluid layer. The chip can be fabricated simply by standard soft lithography using polydimethylsiloxane (PDMS) and glass slide.

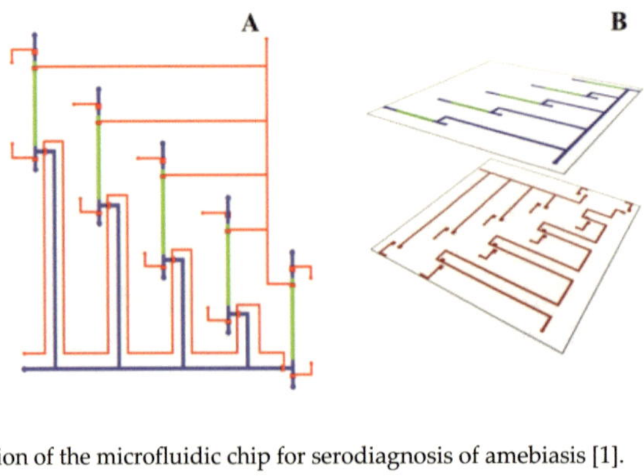

Figure 1. Structure illustration of the microfluidic chip for serodiagnosis of amebiasis [1].

To facilitate the on-chip immune analysis of amebiasis, the channels within the chip upper layer contained the microcolumns (**Figure 2**, green), which were built based on a sieve valve structure that can trap microspheres (C-Ig1 coated beads) so that immune reaction can be carried out within the columns by pushing the reagent and sample suspension passing through the columns, where the antigen bonds with antibody that was on the surface of the microbeads. By opening and closing the valves on both sides of the channel, reagent and wash buffer can be controlled accurately for the whole immune process.

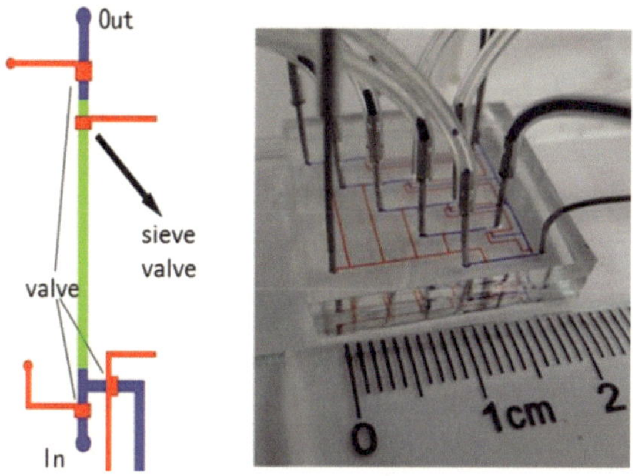

Figure 2. Microcolumn and the microfluidic chip [1].

The fluorescence signals of the immune reactions can be detected by CCD devices. **Figure 3** showed microscope photography of the column within the chip, showing great sensitivity for on-chip detection of amebiasis.

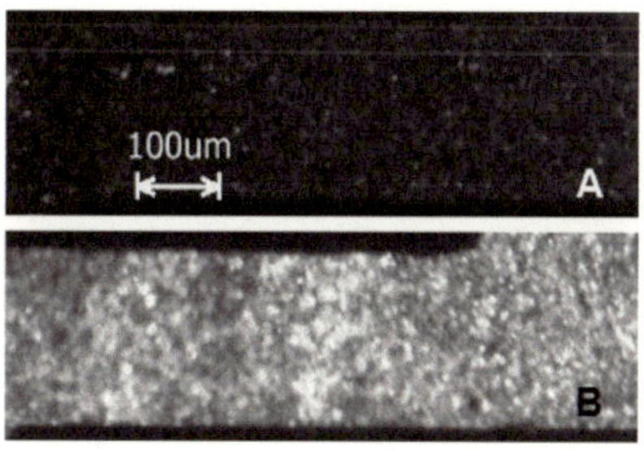

Figure 3. Fluorescence images of the microcolumns [1]. (A) Negative samples. (B) Positive samples.

2.1. Microfluidics for rapid allergy diagnosis

For allergen diagnosis, the UniCAP assay is considered the gold standard in clinical tests. However, serum-specific IgE requires separate analysis that is labor intensive and depends on complicated instruments. As a result, the time and cost expense required for the large-scale allergy survey currently employed deems the method insufficient for many applications. On-chip allergy diagnosis provides many advantages, such as low reagent consumption, short analysis time, simple operation, environmental-friendly process, and high-throughput abilities. The microfluidics can be combined with protein microarray techniques to facilitate large-scale survey and provide a promising platform for clinical applications.

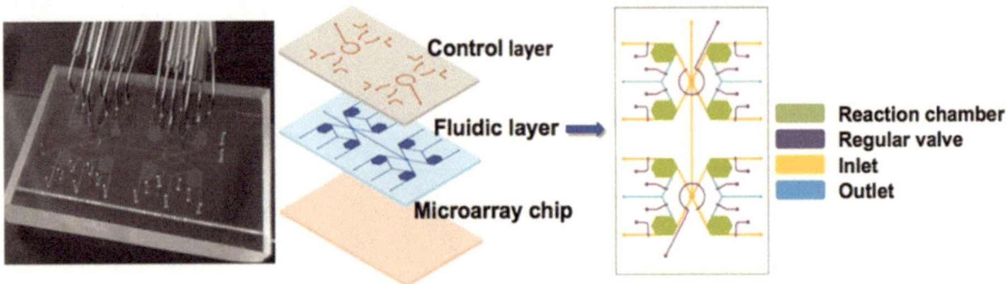

Figure 4. The microfluidic chip for high-throughput allergy diagnosis [2].

Figure 4 shows a three-layer microfluidic chip for high-throughput allergy analysis [2]. The chip was consisted of a control layer, a fluidic layer and a glass slide. Prior to the on-chip analysis, allergens were printed onto the surface of glass slide in triplicate manner using traditional protein microarray technique. The printed slide was then served as the bottom slide of the fluid layer and bonded to the PDMS layers to give a protein hybridization chip. The integrated microvalves within the control layer were used to precisely control reagents inside for the biochemical reaction process.

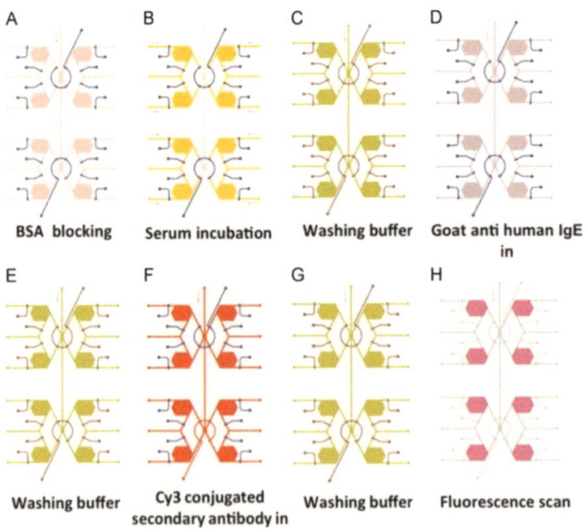

Figure 5. Operation of the microfluidic device for on-chip allergy diagnosis [2].

The operation protocol of the on-chip allergen detections of serum-specific IgE was shown in **Figure 5**. Generally, the hexagonal chambers were filled with blocking buffer containing 3%

BSA, followed by incubating the chip for 1 h at 37°C. After incubation, the eight serum samples (20 × diluted) were loaded into the eight hexagonal hybridization chambers in parallel. Meanwhile, ring-shaped valves within the control layer were closed to prevent cross-contamination. Another incubation at 37°C for 1.5 h was carried out for the bindings. After rinsing the chambers with PBS, goat anti-human IgE antibody was injected. Then, the chip was heated to 37°C for 1 h. Finally, the chip was filled with CY3-labeled secondary antibody IgG. The immune reactions were completed after incubation for 1 h at 37°C. A Luxscan-10K/A microarray scanner was involved to give the fluorescence signals.

Figure 6 shows the obtained fluorescence signals in a single assay. The signals were scanned, and the intensities were calculated for further studies. By combing microarray techniques, the microfluidic device turns into a promising platform for accurate and high-throughput IgE analysis of clinical serum samples, showing potential applications on clinical large-scale screening of allergies.

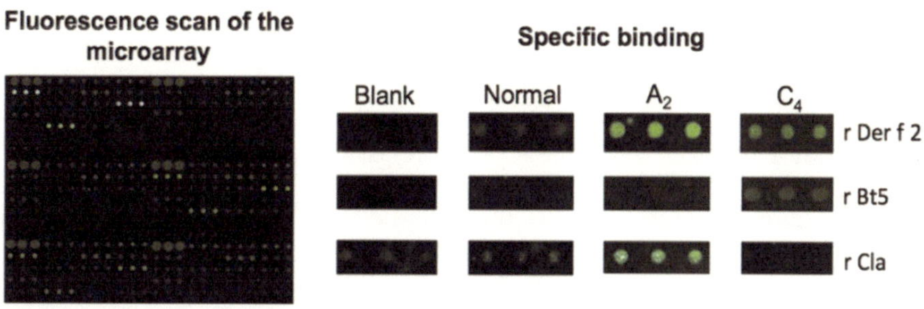

Figure 6. Fluorescence signals on the surface of the glass slide [2].

3. Microfluidics for airborne pathogen analysis (principles and methods)

Airborne pathogens are serious threat to public safety. Due to the lack of technique for rapid detecting airborne pathogens, bacterial transfer by air is very hard to prevent. Although traditional techniques such as Anderson sampler and AGI sampler have been proposed for decades, concentrations of collected pathogens cannot reach the detection limit (LOD) requirement for current bioanalytical methods. Thus, rapid analysis and early warning of airborne pathogen-related diseases is hard to be performed immediately.

We first attempted to used a microfluidic technique to facilitate fast enrichment of airborne pathogens. The microfluidic chip contained a long channel with staggered herringbone mixer (SHM) that was significant for airborne capture with high efficiency. Utilization of the SHM structure dates back to 2002, first proposed by Stroock et al. [3]. The structure was originally designed for mixing of the fluid flowing through microchannels and exhibited impressively high efficiency. Since the SHM possess a large number of ridges along the inner surface of the channel, as fluid flowing through the channels, laminar flow (both liquid and gas) in the chip would be broken. Moreover, the SHM showed high efficiency of mixing fluids in chips and can be simply designed and integrated with standard microfabrication techniques. Because of its benefits, many researchers have utilized the structure in the following decade. In 2013, our group first tried using the SHM structure on airborne bacterial enrichment [4].

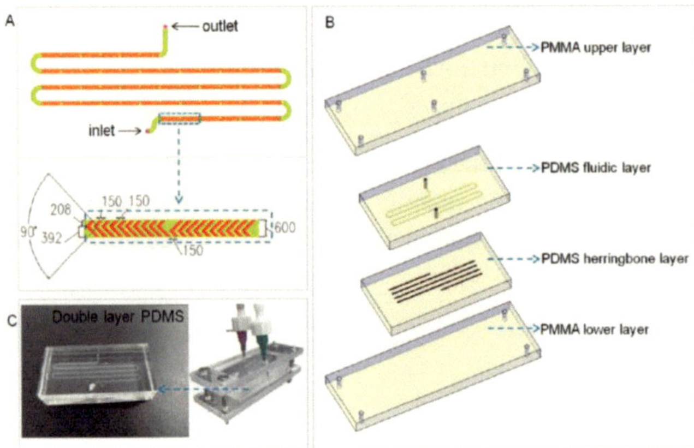

Figure 7. Structure of the microfluidic chip for airborne bacterial capture and enrichment [4].

As shown in **Figure 7**, the double-layer microfluidic chip was fabricated by standard soft lithography using PDMS [5]. The main channel inside the chip contained a standard SHM structure that has a depth of 40 μm, a width of 600 μm and a length of 17.4 cm. Inlet and outlet on each sides of the channel that have diameters of around 1.5 mm were drilled using a puncher. The chip was then clamped lightly with two polymethylmethacrylate (PMMA) plates to reduce air leakage from PDMS wall.

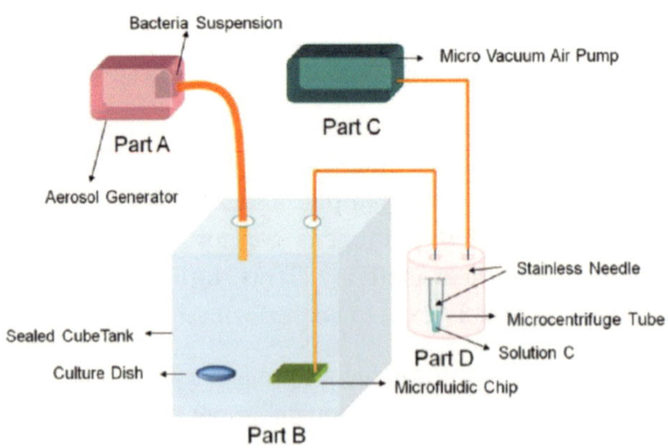

Figure 8. Illustration of the system setup [4].

To simulate bacterial bioaerosol in the natural environment, an aerosol generator and a tank were used to make bacterial bioaerosol. **Figure 8** showed a 125-L glass tank and the setup for the enrichment assay. The microfluidic chip was connected to a microvacuum air pump (HARGRAVES) then put inside the tank. Aqueous bacterial suspension was diluted and then used to generate bioaerosol containing a series of bacterial concentrations.

The flow rate of the microvacuum can be adjusted from 1.0 to 12.0 mL min^{-1}. By drawing the air into the chip, the aerosol passed through the channel very fast. The pumping time can be set from 10 to60 min. The SHM structure helped to break the laminar flow inside the channel, which increased the probability of collision of the airborne bacteria with the inner surface of the channels, so that bacterial cells in the aerosol would hit and attach to the inner surface of the channel wall so as to collect the airborne bacteria.

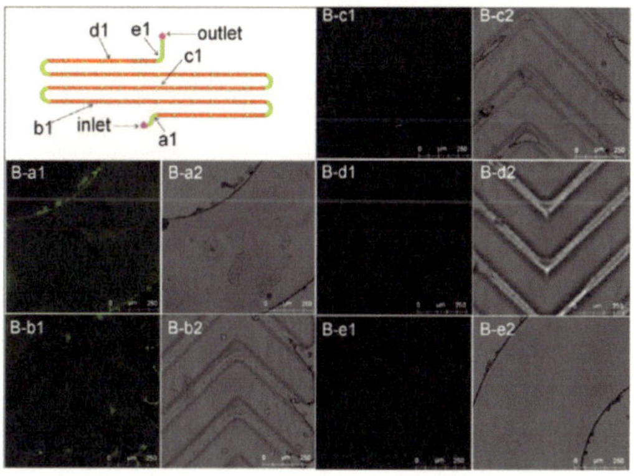

Figure 9. Microscopy photography of fluorescent *E. coli* cells along the channel [4].

To evaluate the enrichment efficiency, GFP-labeled bacteria were used to make the bioaerosol. **Figure 9** showed the fluorescence photography of GFP-labeled *E. coli* cells inside the chip channel after the collection step. Strong fluorescence signals were observed in the front side of the channel, indicating the chip can capture the bacteria with very high efficiency. Along the channel, the GFP signal intensity showed a gradual decrease, indicating that the channel length was enough for airborne bacterial capture with no cells leaking from the chip. Technically, the SHM channel can be build short (around 10–15 cm), which is believed to be long enough for the bacterial capture.

After the enrichment step, a couple of microliters of aqueous media (or lysis buffer) was loaded into the chip. The SHM channel was flushed with ddH_2O. The washed bacterial cells were then moved directly into another microfluidic chip using a micropump for immune or PCR analysis or to bacteria counting using dilution plate or cell culture for further studies.

3.1. Microfluidics for rapid analysis of airborne bacteria (*Escherichia coli, Enterococcus faecalis, Klebsiella pneumoniae, Enterococcus faecalis, Staphylococcus aureus and Citrobacter koseri*)

Polymerase chain reaction (PCR) has been applied to the detection of bacteria for decades. However, PCR often requires DNA purification process which is time-consuming and expensive devices to provide thermal cycles of the reactions to carry out. The defects make the technique not suitable for rapid detecting applications in field. For rapid detections (point-of-care tests) of airborne *Escherichia coli, Enterococcus faecalis, Klebsiella pneumoniae, Enterococcus faecalis, Staphylococcus aureus and Citrobacter koseri,* chip collection followed by on-chip PCR analysis is a very promising way due to the high sensitivity and selectivity of the assay.

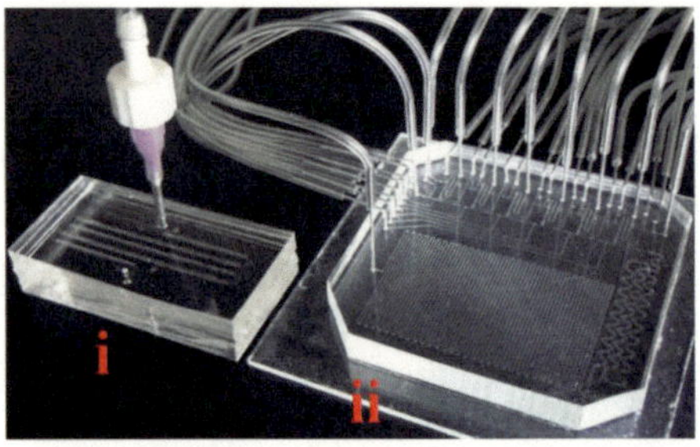

Figure 10. The airborne bacterial enrichment and PCR system [6].

A microfluidic system comprising an airborne bacterial enrichment chip (**Figure 10**, i) and a high-throughput PCR chip (**Figure 10**, ii) is shown in **Figure 10** [6]. The rectangular chip has a length of 5.5 cm and a width of 5.5 cm. The height of the channels inside the chip is 30 μm. To facilitate sample and reaction mixtures inlet and outlet, holes of 650 μm diameter were punched in the chip. The heating process (95 and 55°C) for PCR was provided by two polyimide heating membranes that were assembled beneath the chip.

The 2.5 μl PCR reagent consisting PCR primers for each bacterial target, 0.13 μl bacterial cell lysis products, 0.125 μg BSA, 0.5U ExTaq, 1 × buffer, and 2.5 mM dNTP.

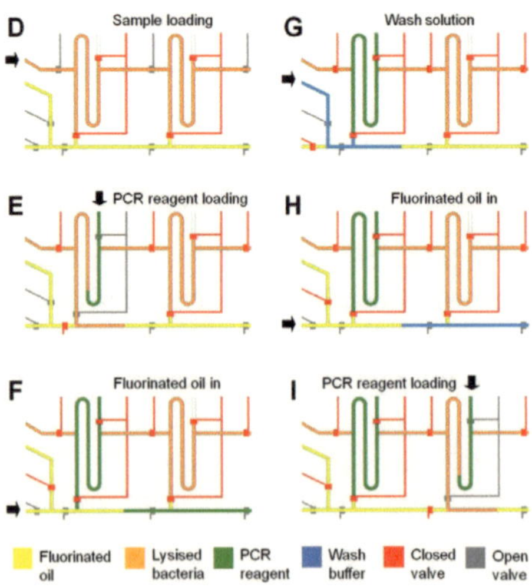

Figure 11. Schematic operating procedures of the high-throughput PCR chip [6].

Figure 11 shows the operating procedures of the PCR chip. After airborne sample collections, the bacterial cell lysis products were washed and injected into the S-shaped sample-loading channels. Next, the channels was isolated via increasing the pressure in the valves, and then the reaction mixtures were loaded into the chip using a micropump, followed by loading fluorinated oil to push the PCR plug to moved inside the channels. To prevent contamination, buffer was loaded to wash the channels inside the chip. Then, fluorinated oil was injected again to push the washing plug to move along the channels. Finally, the following group of reaction mixtures was loaded into an adjacent sample-loading channel. Thus, the six PCRs can be carried out continuously in the chip by repeating the described steps.

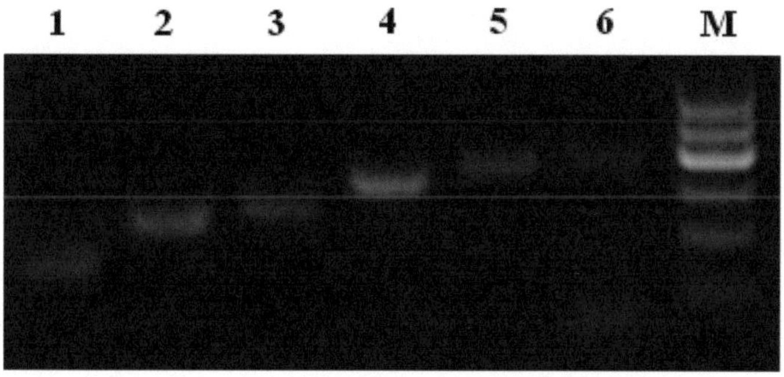

Figure 12. Agarose gel electrophoresis image of the on-chip PCR products [6].

After pushing the reaction mixture plug pass through the temperature zones alternately, the amplified DNA fragments were collected and detected using agarose gel electrophoresis. **Figure 12** shows the PCR produces of airborne (*Escherichia coli, Enterococcus faecalis, Klebsiella pneumoniae, Enterococcus faecalis, Staphylococcus aureus, and Citrobacter koseri*).

3.2. Microfluidics for rapid analysis of airborne *Mycobacterium tuberculosis*

Mycobacterium tuberculosis is considered as the most common cause of tuberculosis infections. The selective analysis of *Mycobacterium tuberculosis* depends on bacteriological immune techniques, while the reagents are expensive and skilled workers are required to run the tests using traditional methods. On the other hand, on-chip immune analysis of *Mycobacterium tuberculosis* has advantages of lower reagent consumption, automatic operation, low detection limit, and shorter assay time.

An integrated microfluidic device for rapid enrichment analysis of airborne *Mycobacterium tuberculosis* was shown in **Figure 13** [7].

The airborne bacterial enrichment part (**Figure 13**, i), as described previously, consisted a SHM structure that facilitates capturing of the airborne *Mycobacterium tuberculosis* in bioaerosol. The following analysis steps of *Mycobacterium tuberculosis* depend on a high-throughput double-layer chip containing control and fluidic layers (**Figure 13**, ii). A standard soft-lithography was used to fabricate PDMS based microfluidic chips.

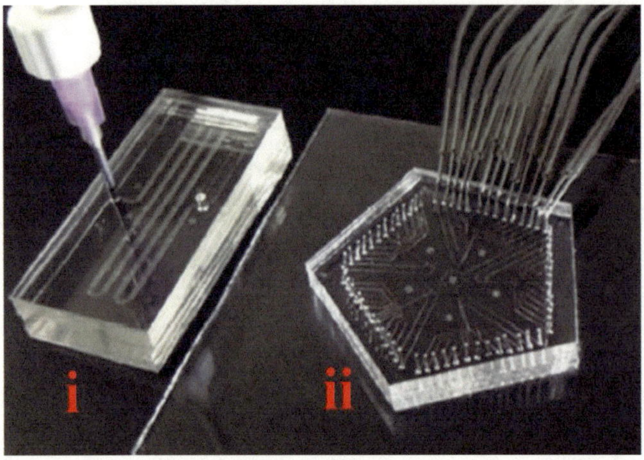

Figure 13. The airborne *Mycobacterium tuberculosis* enrichment analysis chips [7].

On-chip immune analysis targeted on the specific protein Ag85B of *Mycobacterium tuberculosis*. **Figure 14** shows the operations for the on-chip analysis. Sieve valves were built within the channels to form microcolumns [8]. Microspheres pre-coating with protein A and rabbit polyclonal antibody were loaded to work as substrates for capturing the Ag85B. Monoclonal antibody and FITC-conjugated secondary antibody were sequentially injected into the microcolumns to show the signals.

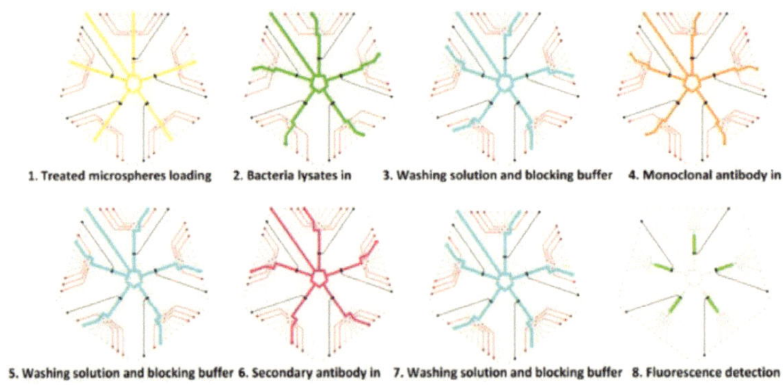

Figure 14. Schematic diagram of operation procedures of the on-chip immune analysis [7].

3.3. Microfluidics for rapid analysis of bacteria in cerebrospinal fluid

For rapid analysis of bacteria in aqueous samples, a promising method is loop-mediated isothermal amplification (LAMP). It is a novel isothermal nucleic acid analysis technique exhibiting high analytical sensitivity with less assay time. The results generated from LAMP amplification are visible to the naked eyes, which makes it a convenient method for rapid diagnostic. On-chip LAMP can be utilized for diagnosis of pathogen infections in cerebrospinal fluid (such like staphylococcus spp.). The reactions require only a couple of microliters of sample and no sophisticated instrument. Plus the aqueous samples can be directly used without a DNA extraction process, providing a robust approach for bacterial detections in field.

Figure 15 shows a three-layer microfluidic chip for cerebrospinal fluid diagnostic [9]. The chip was fabricated from PDMS, where the upper layer controlled the liquid flow within the middle fluid transport layer. To perform four analytical reactions targeting on four different samples, four microchannels for LAMP reactions were fabricated in parallel in the bottom layer of the chip.

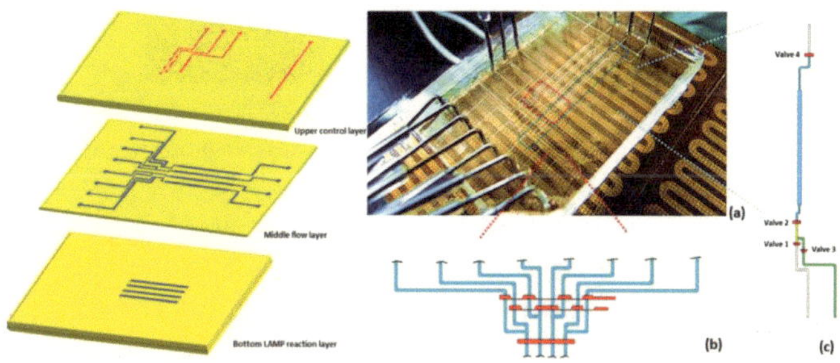

Figure 15. Schematic diagram of the microfluidic chip for LAMP analysis [9].

As shown in **Figure 16**, each unit consists of one sample-loading channel (width 200 μm, depth 30 μm), one lysis chamber (width 200 μm, depth 30 μm), and one amplification chamber (width 400 μm, depth 330 μm). In the microfluidic chip, the channels and chambers were opened and closed by oil valves (**Figure 16**, valve 1–4).

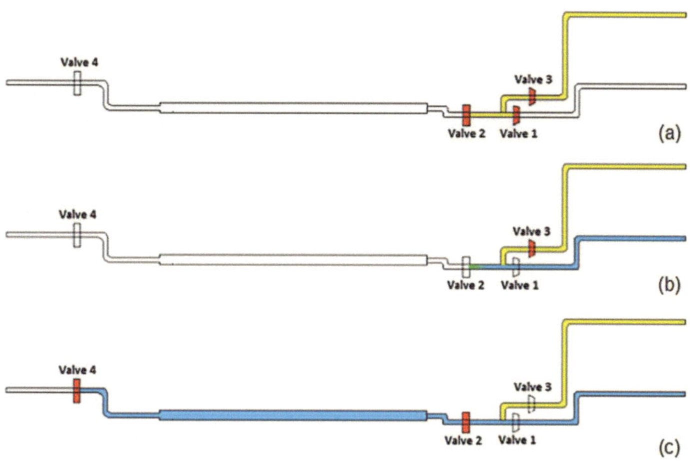

Figure 16. Operation of the microfluidic device for on-chip LAMP [9].

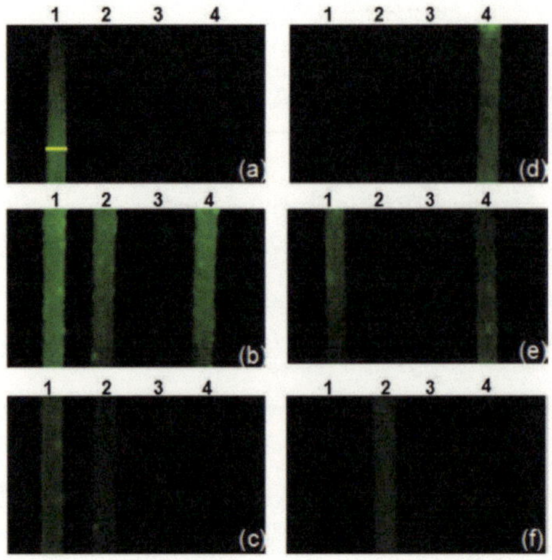

Figure 17. Fluorescence images of LAMP amplifications of clinical cerebrospinal fluid samples [9].

The suspension of aqueous sample mixed with lysis buffer was injected into the channels by a micropump. Valves 1, 2, and 3 were closed to seal the reaction chamber. Then, the chip was heated to 70°C for 30 min as that bacteria in cerebrospinal fluid can be lysed to release DNA. Subsequently, valves 1 and 2 were open. LAMP reagents were injected into the amplification chamber with valve 3 closed. Next, valves 2 and 4 were closed, following by heating the chip to 65°C for 40 min for LAMP amplification. Result signal can be detected under 365 nm UV (**Figure 17**).

Author details

Xiran Jiang[2], Wenwen Jing[1], Lulu Zheng[1], Wang Zhao[1] and Guodong Sui[1*]

*Address all correspondence to: gsui@fudan.edu.cn

1 Shanghai Key Laboratory of Atmospheric Particle Pollution Prevention (LAP[3]), Department of Environmental Science and Engineering, Institute of Biomedical Science, Fudan University, Shanghai, People's Republic of China

2 Department of Biomedical Engineering, Faculty of Electronic Information and Electrical Engineering, Dalian University of Technology, Dalian, People's Republic of China

References

[1] Zhao W, Zhang L, Jinig W, et al. An integrated microfluidic device for rapid serodiagnosis of amebiasis. Biomicrofluidics. 2013;7(1):11101.

[2] Zheng L, Fu Y, Jiang X, et al. Microfluidic system for high-throughput immunoglobulin-E analysis from clinical serum samples. Talanta. 2015;143:83–89.

[3] Stroock AD, Dertinger SK, Ajdari A, et al. Chaotic mixer for microchannels. Science. 2002;295(5555):647–651.

[4] Jing W, Zhao W, Liu S, et al. Microfluidic device for efficient airborne bacteria capture and enrichment. Analytical Chemistry. 2013;85(10):5255–5262.

[5] Whitesides GM, Ostuni E, Takayama S, et al. Soft lithography in biology and biochemistry. Annual Review of Biomedical Engineering. 2001;3:335–373.

[6] Jiang X, Jing W, Zheng Lu, et al. A Continuous-flow high-throughput microfluidic device for airborne bacteria PCR detection. Lab on a Chip. 2014;14:671–676.

[7] Jing W, Jiang X, Zhao W, et al. Microfluidic platform for direct capture and analysis of airborne *Mycobacterium tuberculosis*. Analytical Chemistry. 2014;86(12):5815–5821.

[8] Lee C, Sui G, Elizarov A, et al. Multistep synthesis of a radiolabeled imaging probe using integrated microfluidics. Science. 2005;310(5755):1793–1796.

[9] Yuan H, Zhang J, Jiang X, et al. Microfluidic chip for rapid analysis of cerebrospinal fluid infected with *Staphylococcus aureus*. Analytical Methods. 2014;6:2015–2019.

Chapter 6

Nanotechnology-Based Rapid Diagnostic Tests

Anna Lyberopoulou,
Efstathios P. Efstathopoulos and Maria Gazouli

Additional information is available at the end of the chapter

http://dx.doi.org/10.5772/63908

Abstract

Recently, various nanomaterials are used in order to develop nanotechnology-based rapid diagnostic tests, such as metallic nanoparticles, quantum dots (QDs), silica nanospheres, magnetic nanoparticles, carbon nanotubes (CNTs), silicon nanowires (SiNWs), nanopores, graphene, nanostructured surfaces, and metal films. This novel nanodiagnostic approach will further develop point-of-care (POC) diagnostics and monitoring technologies. Nanobiosensors and microarrays of biosensors can create biochip systems and microfluidic platforms that are the most used nanofabrications for rapid diagnostic tests. These nanoplatforms are constructed for the rapid detection of various diseases or pathogen-specific biomolecules/markers, such as DNA, proteins, whole cells (e.g., circulating tumor cells), and others. The fabrication of small-scale portable devices with the incorporation of nanostructures will offer many advantages in the early detection of various diseases and health-threatening infections by pathogens and in the treatment selection and treatment monitoring. The use of nanostructures in *in vitro* diagnostics gives the opportunity to augment the sensitivity and specificity required in clinical practice, lowers the cost and test time of the assays, and enables portable microfluidic platforms suitable for resource-constrained settings. In this chapter, all the state-of-the-art advantages in this field are discussed, starting with the nanostructures used for the fabrication of nanobiosensors, nanobiosensors arrays, and nanofluidic platforms and the nanodiagnostic use of rapid tests in the detection of pathogens, in cancer management, and glucose monitoring for the management of diabetes disease.

Keywords: Nanotechnology, Nanostructures, point-of-care devices, nanodiagnostics, low-cost and rapid diagnosis

1. Introduction

Nanostructures are used in order to create specific nanodevices for the manipulation of biological systems at the molecular level, and this is what currently defines *nanomedicine*. So far, the integration of nanoparticles with biology has led to the development of diagnostic devices, contrast agents, advanced therapy applications, drug delivery therapy, and imaging approaches. Nanomedicine offers many advantages in everyday clinical practice, taking into consideration the non-invasive approach of the samples used, fast reaction times, specificity, and sensitivity that nanoparticles can offer. Therein, these advantages will lead us closer to the construction of point-of-care mobile nanodevices. In the context of *in vitro* nanodiagnostics, nanotechnology allows the construction of novel sensors and *in vitro* tests, in order to improve the sensitivity of existing tests, to develop new diagnostic test platforms, and to allow point-of-care applications. Thus, *Nanodiagnostics* is defined as the application of nanotechnology for the diagnosis of a dysfunction and/or disease in human, at the earliest stage possible, ideally at the level of a single cell. To achieve this goal, various types of nanotechnologies are currently being explored for use in nanodiagnostic applications. Furthermore, an increase in knowledge in basic research will be seen through the development of microscopic and spectroscopic techniques towards ultrahigh spatial resolution, molecular resolution, and ultrahigh sensitivity that will also help in the creation of advanced *in situ* diagnostics tools. More specifically, nanotechnology-based diagnosis techniques offer great opportunities such as

1. Rapid diagnostic test, potentially in the doctor's office or bedside tests, for the initial diagnosis and treatment selection and treatment monitoring to the doctor/hospital or even at home.

2. The early detection of several diseases in comparison with the efficiency of current techniques. The early detection is very important as it offers the opportunity for earlier diagnosis and thus more therapeutic opportunities.

This chapter summarizes the nanostructures used in nanodiagnostic tests and their applications for the development of rapid diagnostic tests for point-of-care disease management and public health.

2. Nanostructures used in nanodiagnostics

The term *nanostructures* includes materials of <100 nm in size in at least one dimension. There are nanostructures in zero-dimensional (0D), one-dimensional, (1D), and two-dimensional (2D) systems. The dimensions of nanostructures are advantageous for use in diagnostics because they are in the range of the size of various biomolecules such as nucleic acids, small proteins, and viruses. An *in vitro* diagnostic tool is always comprised of an element that is able to identify a biochemical change, activity or concentration of a specific molecule of biological importance in the solution of interest. In a nanobiosensor, a transducer is used to convert this biochemical signal into a quantifiable signal.

The use of nanomaterials in the design of *in vitro* diagnostic systems is offering types of sensors that are characterized by specificity, sensitivity, and robustness. Several kinds of nanomaterials have found attractive applications in *in vitro* diagnostic tests, such as metallic nanoparticles, quantum dots (QDs), silica nanospheres, magnetic nanoparticles, which belong to the zero-dimensional (0D) systems, carbon nanotubes (CNTs), silicon nanowires (SiNWs), nanopores, which belong to the one-dimensional (1D) systems, and graphene, nanostructured surfaces, and metal films, which belong to the two-dimensional (2D) systems.

2.1. Metallic NPs

Metals, especially gold and silver, have the advantageous ability to interact with external fields such as light, radiofrequency, and X-rays. Under a specific wavelength, metals exhibit surface plasmon resonance (SPR), the oscillation of free electrons in a particle's surface; thus, they can successfully be combined with conventional methods such as colorimetry or absorption spectroscopy. A typical example of SPR biosensing consists of the liquid sample part and an immobilized ligand (e.g., an antibody) on an SPR-active gold-coated glass slide. This system can create a thin flow cell in which the sample will be able to flow in the aqueous solution, and when light (visible or near infrared) is projected through the glass slide and onto the gold surface at angles and wavelengths near the SPR condition, the optical reflectivity of the gold changes in a specific way when an actual interaction occurs between the sample and the ligand of the solid phase. The most frequent medical use of these NPs is the rapid tests, for example, pregnancy test kits, where gold nanoparticles are used as a color marker [1]. Moreover, metallic NPs are suitable for surface-enhanced Raman spectroscopy (SERS), since they produce Raman signal. So, when molecules are in close proximity to a metal surface, they exhibit a dramatic augmentation in the electromagnetic field, yielding high Raman intensity. Thus, SERS surface biosensors are usually performed on Ag, Au, or Cu surfaces. SERS is an excellent assay for the sensitive and specific detection of low-concentration molecules, for example, the detection of biomarkers for bacillus spores or the measurement of glucose after the appropriate chemical modifications of the SERS surfaces [2]. Another example is the molecular sentinels, which are comprised of metal NPs decorated with a Raman label-conjugated stem-loop DNA. Thus, when the DNA molecule is in close proximity to the metal surface, the Raman intensity is maintained high. In contrast, in the bound state, there is a disruption of the stem-loop and the Raman label is no longer in close proximity to the metal. This approach was used to detect the *gag* gene of the HIV-1 in PCR amplicons [3] and several single-nucleotide polymorphisms (SNPs) such as *BRCA1* gene of breast cancer, using plasmonic nanoprobes that detach from the Raman tag when the conjugated oligonucleotide is hybridized, thus decreasing the plasmonic effect and change the SERS [4].

2.2. Quantum dots (QDs)

In the field of *in vitro* applications, nanoparticles are mainly used as markers for biomolecules, since they have many optical advantages that make them suitable for several diagnostic assays such as PCR, for the construction of biochips or suitable for multiplexing, conversely to the traditional dyes used in every day clinical practice. To this end, inorganic fluorescent nanoparticles are being investigated such as semiconductor nanoparticles (quantum dots) or nanoparticles-like nanophopsphors, resulting in an increase in sensitivity and specificity and the possible analysis of multiple analytes that offer opportunities of mass production [5].

Quantum dots, semiconductor nanocrystals coated with inorganic materials, are also currently used in the field of basic research of cell biology, and their use in clinical diagnostic tests is already under investigation with great progress as markers, especially in image-guided techniques, and at the same time, some nanobiochip platforms are already in the market. More importantly, QDs are very efficient donors of energy compared to traditional organic dyes, especially dye acceptors in FRET-based assays (fluorescence resonance energy transfer) [6].

2.3. Silica nanospheres

Just like QDs, inorganic dye-loaded silica particles are characterized by good photostability, sharp emission peaks, and long-lasting fluorescence lifetimes. They are appropriate for dispersion aqueous solutions, due to their hydrophilic surface. They are usually used to conjugate optical labels in order to increase the detection signal, such as organic or inorganic dye molecules (lanthanide-based and ruthenium-based) [7].

2.4. Magnetic NPs

Last but not least is the use of *supermagnetic iron oxide nanoparticles (SPIOs)*, which are used for magnetic separation in several immunomagnetic applications such as cell sorting, nucleic acid extraction, purification, and detection of pathogens, cancer cells, and generally rare populations in a solution/sample [8].

2.5. Carbon nanotubes or nanopores (CNTs–CNPs)

There are a variety of challenges associated with the flow of liquids through carbon *nanotubes* and *nanopores*. These are small electrically insulated tubes or pores which can detect a single molecule when this passes through the tube or pore. The molecule's detection is based on the change of the ionic current of the electrolyte solution containing the molecules of interest, which results in a change of the electrical current (translocation event signal) [7]. The incorporation of biochips and nanofluidics with nanopores or nanotubes will be able to replace the existing sequencing approaches of DNA in the clinical practice, as each DNA base has unique molecular structure and thus a unique translocation event signal. To this aim, nanofluidic devices are developed that employ multiple measurements on single molecules to enhance the ability to size DNA molecules. Techniques to integrate membranes contain nanopores into microfluidic devices, which decrease noise and enable the design of networks containing nanopores.

2.6. Silicon nanowires (SiNWs)

Nanowires are currently believed to be unique and advantageous for the construction of a nanobiosensing device. Nanowires are nanoscale channels through which current is passed and can be constructed from carbon nanotubes, metal oxides or silicon, and they require high temperatures to be synthesized and are usually prepared on silicon wafers. Antibodies are usually used as detectors in the surface of the nanowire. Antibodies interact with the biological target of interest, and the conformational change results in a change in the current that passes through the nanowire, allowing a sensitive and specific detection. The use of nanowires in an array mode, where different antibodies are conjugated to each nanowire, allows the mass detection of different types of disease or the creation of a personalized molecular profile in one type of disease [7].

2.7. Graphene, metal films and nanostructured surfaces

Graphene, metal films, and nanostructured surfaces are all in the class of 2D nanostructures which are structures with one dimension of ~100 nm in size. Their incorporation in nanodiagnostic is their use as racks in order to conjugate and immobilize ligands for targeted binding when the sample comes across them. They usually are sheets of a certain nanomaterial, which have special properties different from that of the corresponding bulk material. For example, metal films exhibit the same advantages with metal NPs, for example, the SPR effect, and thus, they are used in the construction of label-free SPR biosensors. As for nanostructured surfaces, they are in reality electrodes with their surface linked with nanotubes or nanoparticles. Finally, graphene will offer great sensitivity in rapid diagnostic tests, since it is an incredibly stable one-layer 2D surface of carbon atoms with unique optical and conductive properties [7].

3. Nanotechnology-on-a-chip or nanofluidics

A nanobiochip is comprised of integrated biomolecules or biologically active artificial structures which are usually smaller than that of cell's. The chip contains microarrays, which are minitest sites, on a solid surface, and this allows for multiple tests to be carried out simultaneously. Therefore, identification of a specific molecular signature, which will be unique to the diagnosis, can be done through thousands of biochemical reactions being performed on the nanobiochip [9, 10].

The identification and quantification of a variety of molecules will be permitted through the combination of nanotechnologies, such as nanofluids and nanobiosensors, with biochips, and this will lead to the generation of future *in vitro* diagnostic chip-based devices. Nanofluidic structures have small fluidic conducts which means they are automatically applied in situations where you have extremely small quantities of the sample. This includes Coulter counting, analytical separations and determinations of biomolecules, such as proteins and DNA and facile handling of mass-limited samples. Lab-on-a-chip structures comprise one of the more promising tools of nanofluidics. The advance and production of lab-on-chip devices for PCR and other related techniques mean that nanofluidics have had a substantial impact in biotechnology, medicine, and clinical diagnostics. In nanofluidics, a chamber of up to a few hundred nanometers in size contains a liquid sample which is then manipulated and analyzed. As the volume of the samples are so small, this allows for a substantial reduction in the amount of sample needed for the analysis as well as allowing for the advantages of laminar flow conditions, high surface to volume rations, low concentrations, molecular confinement, and low heat capacity to be used. On the other hand, nanofluidics also generates new challenges in the device design and manufacture, the accurate control of flow and mixing, and the sensitivity of molecular detection, and they are starting to be used in many diagnostic and analytical devices [10, 11].

An *in vitro* simple detection system can therefore be established, which allows hundreds of cantilever biosensors to be used simultaneously on the same array. A lab-on-a-chip device could be produced through additional advances of this technique which include the complete integration with fluidic handling system, other analytical techniques and signal extraction electronic. The initial proposition, by Berger et al., was for a "laboratory-on-a-tip" which described the potential combination of cantilever sensors with atomic force microscopy (AFM). In this proposed technique, a cantilever with a tip could examine and detect with nanometer resolution where the biochemical analysis is executed. Thus, in conclusion, an alternative PCR which has the potential to replace microarray detection techniques is offered through cantilever nanobiosensing for the identification of SNPs, oncogenes, viruses, bacteria, and a variety of other pathogens. Additionally, the most common *in vitro* application of SPR biosensor chip devices is defining the affinity parameters of biomolecular interactions, where a sensorgram is used to report the association and dissociation of the ligand and its binding partner, which is added once the ligand has been immobilized on the sensor chip. There are numerous advantages of using this technique in comparison with conventional methods for affinity measurement, and these include little material being required, it is very quick, and finally, no tracer is needed for labeling. The expanding field of proteomics has seen the most recent developments in SPR where it is combined with matrix-assisted laser desorption/ ionization time of flight mass spectrometry (MALDI-TOF), and this permits the study of biomolecular interactions between molecules of which at least one is known. The interacting molecule cannot always be identified when a variety of proteins is used within the interaction study. However, using the MALDI-TOF technique allows you to determine the molecule that interacts with the sensor from the mixture [10, 11].

4. Applications of nanotechnology in *in vitro* nanodiagnostics

Up to now, nanostructures are successfully incorporated to *in vitro* diagnostics for the construction of nanobiosensors and *in vitro* rapid diagnostic tests mainly in order to improve existing tests and make them more effective or create innovative diagnostic test approaches that will be able to be incorporated in point-of-care applications of every day clinical practice. Nanodiagnostic applications are currently focused on two main approaches, such as the use of nanoparticles as biomarkers and the development of novel nanosensors that incorporate various nanostructures, such as carbon nanotubes, lateral nanostructures or nanothin surface layers via labeled nanosensors or label-free nanosensors. With the use of *in vitro* diagnostic tests based on nanotechnology, various clinical and research fields will be improved such as genotyping techniques, immunohistochemistry assays, detection of biomarkers, early cancer detection, and others. Below, we are going to describe some of these applications.

4.1. Nanosensors for glucose monitoring

The management of diabetes disease, besides the great progress in the maintenance of insulin, is still intriguing. In the current clinical practice, diabetes patients need to tolerate tandem blood samples in order to monitor blood glucose and therefore minimize the possibility of hyper- or hypoglycemia, together with the aftermaths. Thus, it is still now an essential task to design a management approach for the monitoring of blood glucose that is non-invasive, fast, and sensitive. The use of nanotechnology for the fabrication of a rapid and portable diagnostic test offers the aforementioned advantages. However, it is difficult task to design the ideal test, since the ideal biosensor has to be small, low-cost, with simple function, accurate in the measurement and of course portable. Furthermore, this future test will have to minimize the blood volume needed for the test and the possible contaminations and to assure the accuracy of the measurement. Even further, an implantable microfluidics biosensor could provide a more accurate management of *in vivo* glucose monitoring and insulin administration. Barone et al. [12] used solution-phase optical single-walled CNTs (SWCNTs) sensors which have a tunable near-infrared (NIR) emission that responds to changes in the local dielectric function, but remains stable to permanent photobleaching. SWCNTs are integrated with beta-D-glucose sensing as a model system; for example, they are conjugated with glucose oxidase, an enzyme that degrades glucose molecules and ferricyanide a molecule that takes electrons from the NTs, quenching their capacity to glow under NIR. In order to test the *in vivo* capacity of the nanosensors, they implanted them in situ in a human skin tissue sample and excited with NIR. The results demonstrated that the higher the glucose concentration, the greater the fluorescence. Thus, the nanosensors were found able to modulate their emission in response to the adsorption of specific biomolecules, suggesting that nanoparticle optical sensors are an attractive solution for glucose monitoring [12]. However, such techniques that use glucose consumption turned out to have many disadvantages regarding the continuous glucose monitoring. Therefore, technique based on competitive affinity binding of glucose and subcutaneously implanted enzymatic electrochemical detection is being recently a very attractive approach, since they can be highly stable and low drift. For example, the use of a polysaccharide solution such as dextran conjugated to a glucose-binding protein such as concanavalin A (Con A), which competitively binds glucose leading to reversible de-cross linking of the dextran–Con A complex. In the unbound state, the changes in the fluorescence or viscosity of the solution can be detected. Alternatively, synthetic glucose-responsive polymers have been recently fabricated from various research groups in order to substitute Con A, which is found to be cytotoxic and fast degradable. Huang et al. [13] fabricated a biocompatible, glucose-specific polymer (PAA-ran-PAAPBA) in order to create a sensor based on the sensing principle of the viscosity detection changes due to affinity binding between glucose and (PAA-ran-PAAPBA). Microelectromechanical system (MEMS) technology was incorporated for the fabrication of the sensor device that allowed long-term continuous glucose monitoring [14]. The device uses a magnetically responsive vibrating Parylene polymer microcantilever as sensing element, situated in a microchamber, which was filled by PAA-ran-PAAPBA. Glucose passes through the membrane and binds reversibly to (PAA-ran-PAAPBA) polymer, causing a viscosity alteration in the solution. The MEMS device was suggested as a subcutaneously implanted sensor for stable and reliable continuous monitoring of glucose in practical diabetes management [13].

Recently, a type of miniaturized sensors called optodes has attracted the scientists' attention. Nano-optodes consist of a chemical that responds to an analyte, a polymer to immobilize the chemical transducer and instrumentation (optical fiber, light source, detector, and other electronics) [15]. They can be integrated with several optical measurement schemes such as reflection, absorption, evanescent wave, luminescence (fluorescence and phosphorescences) that is the most popular methodology, chemiluminescence and surface plasmon resonance. Balaconis et al. [16] used nanofiber fluorescent nano-optodes in order to measure the dynamic changes of glucose concentrations based on the competitive binding between a hydrophobic boronic acid recognition molecule, a chromophore and glucose. The concentration change of glucose in the membrane was monitored by measuring the change of the optical signal. Nano-optodes are proven to be functional both *in vitro* and *in vivo* and to be very sensitive, since they can detect even small molecules [15, 16].

4.2. Detection of bacteria and viruses

Nowadays, pathogen detection is performed using very sensitive techniques such as ELISA, PCR, and sequencing techniques. However, the aforementioned techniques are considered very expensive; they require excessive sample preparation and have long validation times with no early response; and they need expertise personnel to perform the test. Therefore, the advantageous optical, magnetic, electrical, and catalytic characteristics of nanomaterials can offer faster, more sensitive, specific, and cheaper diagnostic assays that no experts will be needed for their use, in order to detect microbial pathogenesis. Pathogens express on their membranes various molecules such as glyco-, lipoproteins, glycopeptides, carbohydrates, and lipids. Thus, nanotechnology usually uses antibodies as targeting ligands for the development of various immunoassays. For example, gold and silver NPs have been broadly used for conjugation with affinity ligands, finding attractive applications as chemical sensors or even further for the generation of nanoscale arrays of pathogen-targeting ligands. Moreover, NPs can also be conjugated with specific oligonucleotides sequences that bind pathogen nucleic acid sequences to generate colorimetric changes. Other nanoparticles including fluorescent QDs and CNTs have been used in various applications including DNA detection and the development of immunoassays for the detection of bacteria and viruses. Besides NPs based-assays, miniaturized microfluidic system or lab-on-a-chip (LOC) is a futuristic and attractive field of research for accurate and point of care management of microbial infections.

Very recently, Wu et al. [17] fabricated a Microbead Quantum-dots Detection System (MQDS) in order to identify and measure target DNAs of pathogenic microorganisms and substitute PCR amplifications. All reporter probes and internal control probes were conjugated with quantum dots that fluoresce at different emission wavelengths using the click reaction, in order to monitor the binding process by flow cytometry [17]. Zhang et al. [18] created an innovative microfluidic microbead array with QDs tags for HBV genotyping. This method detected *in vitro*-transcribed RNA in serum samples with increased sensitivity of 1000 copies/mL of HBV virus. Thus, they were able to create a QDs-based biochip of high specificity and sensitivity for virus genotyping based on DNA hybridization. This microfluidic device managed to incorporate the microarray technology with the advantages of QDs when used as fluorescent agents and thus suggested a microfluidic approach for the highly sensitive detection of virus DNA of analysis with the use of small sample amount and fast detection time [18]. Moreover, Fu et al. [19] used Raman reporter-labeled AuNPs as SERS nanotags which target the HIV-1 DNA marker. The oligonucleotide-conjugated AuNPs were anchored in user-friendly lateral flow (LF) strips that have been extensively used for point-of-care (POC) self-diagnostics. They managed to analyze HIV-1 DNA with high sensitivity by monitoring the characteristic of Raman peak intensity of the DNA-conjugated AuNPs. The detection limit of these SERS-based lateral flows was observed to be at least 1000 times more sensitive compared to colorimetric or fluorescent detection methods. These results demonstrate the potential feasibility of the proposed SERS-based lateral flow assay to quantitatively detect a wide range of genetic diseases with high sensitivity [19]. Tsang et al. [20] used upconversion nanoparticles (UNPs), based on the upconversion phenomenon where the absorption of photons results in a shorter wavelength emission of light compared to the excitation wavelength. So far, the most common UNPs are the lanthanide Yb^{3+} to Er^{3+} ions as used in this study, where Yb^{3+} ions have the ability to convert to Er^{3+} ions under NIR light and emit at green, visible wavelengths. These UNPs are linked with AuNPs which are conjugated with oligonucleotide probes (AuNPs) targeting Ebola virus oligonucleotide, and this nanocomposite is anchored on a nanoporous alumina (NAAO) membrane. Taking into consideration that Ebola outbreaks are currently of great concern, it is essential to investigate the feasibility of detection nanodevices of into low-cost, rapid, and with ultrasensitive detection of various pathogens, especially epidemic viruses [20].

Besides DNA, antimicrobial peptides (AMPs) are promising affinity agents for the development of biosensors due to the possibility of recognizing a various pathogenic biomarkers (bacteria, fungi, toxins, viruses), in order to design biosensors that exhibit more specificity and sensitivity regarding the detection limits. In the bound state, the biosensor can be evaluated via electrochemical impedance and fluorescence spectroscopies. Mannoor et al. [21] fabricated an array electrobiosensor functionalized with the AMP magainin I on the surface of AuNPs, in order to detect pathogenic bacteria. When the specific reaction occurs between magainin I and the sample, dielectric alterations of the surface's properties are detected, a change that allows the selective detection of pathogenic Gram-negative bacteria *E. coli* and *Salmonella typhimurium* related to the non-pathogenic *E. coli* and the Gram-positive species *Listeria monocytogenes* [21]. It is also possible to use synthetic peptides in order to maximize the selectivity like Lillehoj et al. [22] who designed a microelectromechanical sensor using two synthetic peptides (C16G2cys and G10KHc) for the detection of *Streptococcus mutans* and *Pseudomonas aeruginosa.* On the other hand, Cho and Irudayaraj [23], proposed an *in situ* immuno-AuNP network-based ELISA biosensor to detect pathogens with high sensitivity. The *in situ* ELISA biosensor was able to detect *E. coli* and *S. typhimurium* in real sample conditions within 2 h of inoculation pathogens at extremely low concentrations.

As already mentioned, 2D nanostructures can offer great sensitivity in rapid diagnostic tests. Mevold et al. [24] used graphene–PDDA nanosheets absorbed with AuNPs. PDDA is a homopolymer for the dispersibility of graphene, since it charges positively the graphene and protects the solution from the aggregation of graphene. The positive charge of AuNPs/graphene–PDDA nanosheets serves to easily capture the negative charge of *Staphylococcus aureus* and small molecules (adenine) for SERS rapid detection [24]. Moreover, Li et al. [25] aimed to detect foodborne pathogens, such as *Escherichia coli* O157:H7, *Salmonella enterica, Vibrio cholera,* and *Campylobacter jejuni,* all at the same time using multiplex PCR and magnetic nanoparticle probes (MNPs). The MNPs were conjugated with streptavidin, immobilized in an oligonucleotide array and used in order to visualize the hybridization between the oligonucleotide array and the 5′ biotinylated single-strand PCR products. Interestingly, the signal could be easily detected by naked eye or a microscope. The streptavidin–MNPs microarray detected 316 foodborne pathogens/mL and thus suggested as a sensitive, specific, and easy-to-use tool for the fast detection of foodborne pathogens in a modestly equipped laboratory, being an attractive approach for future rapid diagnostic tests [25].

4.3. Nanotechnology in cancer diagnosis

The incorporation of nanotechnology in cancer diagnosis is essential, since early detection of the disease can improve the chances of treatment. In addition, the reduction of the needed time for the nanotest will lead in more precise decision-making in every day clinical practice and treatment costs.

Up to now, several nanomaterials, such as AuNPs, semiconductor II–VI QDs, silicon nanowires (SNWs), carbon CNTs, and graphene, have been used in order to detect various cancer markers (proteins/peptides or DNA/RNA) in a sensitive and specific manner, especially when used for the construction of high-performance nanobiosensors. For instance, FET-SNWs have been used for the detection of several prostate cancer biomarkers, such as prostate-specific antigen (PSA) at the level of fg/ml of PSA for monitoring prostate cancer and predicting the risk of early biochemical relapse and the prostate biomarker 8-hydroxydeoxyguanosine (8-OHdG) by using a SNWs functionalized with antibodies against 8-OHdG [26]. PSA, prostate-specific membrane antigen, platelet factor-4, and interleukin-6 prostate cancer biomarkers have also been detected by electrochemical NTs [27, 28].

Furthermore, using a nanowire technology (nCounter Analysis System), ribonucleic acid (RNA) expression levels of cancer-testis antigens (CTAs) have been measured, as biomarkers for aggressive prostate cancer. This nanowire technology offers the possibility of a sensor chip, is able to simultaneously detect more than one of cancer marker, and measures a panel of biomarkers related to a specific cancer type and/or individual, thus contributing to the personalization of cancer diagnosis [29]. Lee et al. [30] developed a nanowire substrate-enabled laser-scanning imaging combined with flow cytometry for the isolation and quantitation of circulating tumor cells from a human lung carcinoma sample mixture of tumor cells and leukocytes.

Interestingly, CNTs and SNWs have been utilized for detection of various volatile organic compounds (VOCs) in breath samples of lung and gastric cancer patients, respectively [31]. Thus, Tran et al. [32] constructed a portable read-out NWs on-a-chip device, by the addition of a complementary metal-oxide semiconductor (CMOS) on FET-SiNWs, creating a nanoplatform that could detect ALCAM in serum at a detection limit of 15.5 pg/ml, in <30 min. Besides cancer biomarker detection, FET-SiNWs and zinc oxide nanowires (ZnONWs) have been used to detect ssDNA and mi-RNAs related to the initiation and progression of various cancer types [33].

Just like other nanobiosensors, nanocantilevers were demonstrated to be able to detect PSA at low levels (0.2 ng/ml–60 μg/ml) for the detection of prostate cancer. Huber et al. [34] used microcantilever arrays to detect BRAFV600E mutation nanomechanically without amplification, from total RNA samples isolated from malignant melanoma cells. Wang et al. [35] fabricated a new cantilever array-based biosensor based on MEMS for the detection of alpha-fetoprotein (AFP), a liver cancer biomarker, with high accuracy, while Liu et al. [36] detected the same biomarker for hepatocellular carcinoma at the level of ng/ml, using a resonant microcantilever electromagnetic resonance-exciting and piezoresistive read-out elements on-chip integrated, in order to measure frequency-shift versus specific-adsorbed mass.

So far, nanostructures such as QDs, AuNPs, and superparamagnetic NPs have been the most successfully incorporated in *in vitro* diagnostic applications, due to their potential to be functionalized by several biomolecules (antibodies, oligonucleotides) against the target biomolecules of interest. In the field of *in vitro* diagnostics, nanoparticles are mainly used as markers for biomolecules. On the other hand, conventional fluorescent dyes already used in medical laboratory tests, in PCR assays, and in biochips are not photostable or suitable for multiplexing. Jokerst et al. [37] used semiconductor nanoparticle QDs combined with a microfluidic biosensor for the multiplex quantitation of cancer biomarkers such as carcinoembryonic antigen (CEA), cancer antigen 125 (CA125), and Her-2/Neu (C-erbB-2) in serum and whole saliva specimens. This QD nanobiochip assay system resulted in a 30 times signal amplification, compared with standard molecular fluorophores [37]. Moreover, supermagnetic iron oxide nanoparticles are used, integrated with applications such as cell sorting, nucleic acid extraction and purification for the detection and isolation of circulating tumor cells of several types of cancer such as colorectal, lung, and breast cancer [38–40]. Besides circulating tumor cells, recently circulating extracellular vesicles and exosomes are demonstrated to serve as cancer biomarkers. Kanwar et al. [41] fabricated a microfluidic device (ExoChip) in polydimethylsiloxane (PDMS) and conjugated with antibodies against CD63, overexpressed mainly in exosomes. The ExoChip was able to measure fluorescent-carbocyanine-dyed exosomes from pancreatic cancer patients, compared to those from healthy subjects. Overall, the aim of this study was to suggest a novel approach for cancer molecular profiling that can be applied in various cancer types. Specifically, they managed to create an exosomal-microRNA profiling that could enable the future molecular screening and diagnosis of human cancers [41].

5. Discussion and future perspectives

Up to now, the incorporation of nanostructures in medicine is offering the development of diagnostic tools of high sensitivity, advantageous contrast agents compared to traditional dyes already in use, novel personalized treatment approaches, and drug delivery vehicles. Taking into consideration small-sized sample volumes, fast reaction times, specificity and sensitivity of nanosystems, in the near future they will be able to bring mobile testing devices into every day clinical practice. Regarding *in vitro* nanodiagnostics, nanotechnology allows the construction of high sensitive nanosensors and *in vitro* tests to develop new diagnostic nanoplatforms and to allow point of care applications. Many of the technologies described in this chapter are demonstrated to be versatile; for instance, they are suitable for DNA and protein detection, and they detect very few pathogens, such as bacteria and viruses, or molecules such as low concentration of glucose that would not be detected with conventional techniques. The incorporation of nanotechnology in medicine will lead to the development of rapid diagnostic tests, which will result in the improvement of clinical decision-making and treatment costs. For example, rapid diagnostic nanotests offer early detection of disease such as cancer improving this way the possibilities of treatment.

NPs are the most versatile material for developing diagnostics, since they can be conjugated with various agents and serve as tags or labels. Thus far, there are several efforts in the way in order to develop nanoparticle-based systems for disease detection. Nanosphere, Inc. has launched the Verigene system which uses AuNPs. Verigene system is a molecular diagnostic system for rapid diagnostic evaluation that enables rapid treatment decisions regarding targeted therapy for various infections in bloodstream, respiratory tract, and gastrointestinal tract. The technology can also be applied in the future for other life-threatening diseases such as cardiovascular, autoimmune diseases, and cancer. T2 Biosystems developed T2MR, a diagnostic detection method that uses miniaturized magnetic resonance technology in order to measure how water molecules react under magnetic fields. The T2MR technology platform offers a fast, simple, and sensitive alternative to existing diagnostic methodologies and uses magnetic nanoparticles to identify proteins, nucleic acids, and other materials. T2MR technology enables low limit of detection, as low as 1 cell/mL, compared to the 100–1000 cell/mL required by PCR-based *in vitro* diagnostics. Up to now, T2Candida is in clinical trials and can identify the five clinically relevant species of Candida with 99.4% specificity and 91.1% sensitivity, directly from whole blood which enables physicians to initiate appropriate therapy on the same day. All other FDA-cleared Candida diagnostics require a blood culture to determine the Candida species, which takes up to 6 days for species identification or negative result. On the other hand, the conjugation of virus-specific antibodies in AuNPs can enable the rapid diagnosis of flu virus. The AuNPs–antibodies complex targets the virus in a way that larger AuNPs-virus aggregates are formed. Subsequently, in the presence of light, the sample leads to an increase of the reflected light due to these aggregates, allowing a much faster

http://dx.doi.org/10.5772/63908

validation and virus detection than with the tests currently used. The same notion of the formation of aggregates around the biomolecule of interest is used for the fast and specific detection of various diseases.

Currently, QD technology is the most broadly employed nanotechnology for diagnostic developments, especially for cancer management. The only concern about QDs is the *in vivo* toxicity. However, researchers suggest the use of QDs composed of silicon, which is believed to be less toxic than the cadmium contained in many QDs.

Regarding circulating cancer cell detection, researches have recently published the NanoFlare genetic-based technology that enables the detection of living circulating tumor cells in bloodstream. A NanoFlare is designed to enter cells and to hybridize with cancer-specific oligonucleotide sequences. NanoFlare has a great advantage, such as all nanoparticles due to their size: the fact that they can enter inside the cell gives the opportunity of the use of various biomolecules that are present inside the cell and not only markers anchored on the cell's surface. So when NanoFlare attaches to the cancer-specific target into the cell, a reporter "flare" is released that produces a detectable fluorescent signal.

Nanosensors and blood sensors capable of detecting multiple pathogens or chemical compounds are one such example. Point-of-care diagnostics are possible with nanosensors and also an attractive technology towards point-of-care diagnosis that will be easy for the patient to use at home and will enable the integration of diagnostics with therapeutics and the development of personalized treatment approaches. Blood sensors, especially cantilevers arrays, are characterized by important advantages since the technology of nanomechanical detection requires no labels and/or external probes, and optical excitation and is rapid, highly specific, sensitive, and portable. The above give the opportunity to detect pathogens or molecules in blood samples and are a great example of future point-of-care diagnostic tools. Furthermore, the upper goal regarding the construction of diagnostic biochips will be the miniaturization of the biosensor chips to range of "nano"-dimensions. Thus, the use of nanotechnology in rapid diagnostic tests will lead to devices with nanodimensions, sensitive, easy to use, and non-expensive in order to allow direct signal observation, manipulation, analysis, and result validation of a single biological molecule from a single cell. This offers new opportunities and provides powerful tools in the fields of genomics, proteomics, molecular diagnostics, and high-throughput screening.

Author details

Anna Lyberopoulou[1,2], Efstathios P. Efstathopoulos[1,2] and Maria Gazouli[1,2*]

*Address all correspondence to: mgazouli@med.uoa.gr

1 Department of Basic Medical Sciences, Laboratory of Biology, National and Kapodistrian University of Athens, Athens, Greece

2 Department of Radiology, Medical School, National and Kapodistrian University of Athens, Athens, Greece

References

[1] Majdalawieh A, Kanan MC, El-Kadri O, Kanan SM. Recent advances in gold and silver nanoparticles: synthesis and applications. J Nanosci Nanotechnol. 2014 Jul;14(7):4757–80. Review.

[2] Kong K, Kendall C, Stone N, Notingher I. Raman spectroscopy for medical diagnostics —from in-vitro biofluid assays to in-vivo cancer detection. Adv Drug Deliv Rev. 2015 Jul 15;89:121–34.

[3] Wabuyele MB, Vo-Dinh T. Detection of human immunodeficiency virus type 1 DNA sequence using plasmonics nanoprobes. Anal Chem. 2005 Dec 1;77(23):7810–5.

[4] Wabuyele MB, Yan F, Vo-Dinh T. Plasmonics nanoprobes: detection of single-nucleotide polymorphisms in the breast cancer BRCA1 gene. Anal Bioanal Chem. 2010 Sep; 398(2):729–36.

[5] Mukherjee A, Shim Y, Myong Song J. Quantum dot as probe for disease diagnosis and monitoring. Biotechnol J. 2016 Jan;11(1):31–42.

[6] Shamirian A, Ghai A, Snee PT. QD-based FRET probes at a glance. Sensors (Basel). 2015 Jun 4;15(6):13028–51.

[7] Choi S, Tripathi A, Singh D. Smart nanomaterials for biomedics. J Biomed Nanotechnol. 2014 Oct;10(10):3162–88. Review.

[8] Singh D, McMillan JM, Kabanov AV, Sokolsky-Papkov M, Gendelman HE. Bench-to-bedside translation of magnetic nanoparticles. Nanomedicine (Lond). 2014 Apr;9(4): 501–16.

[9] Su W, Gao X, Jiang L, Qin J. Microfluidic platform towards point-of-care diagnostics in infectious diseases. J Chromatogr A. 2015 Jan 16;1377:13–26.

[10] Xia D, Yan J, Hou S. Fabrication of nanofluidic biochips with nanochannels for applications in DNA analysis. Small. 2012 Sep 24;8(18):2787–801.

[11] Xu Y, Jang K, Yamashita T, Tanaka Y, Mawatari K, Kitamori T. Microchip-based cellular biochemical systems for practical applications and fundamental research: from microfluidics to nanofluidics. Anal Bioanal Chem. 2012 Jan;402(1):99–107.

[12] Barone PW, Baik S, Heller DA, Strano MS. Near-infrared optical sensors based on single-walled carbon nanotubes. Nat Mater. 2005;4:86–92.

[13] Huang X, Li S, Schultz JS, Wang Q, Lin Q. A MEMS affinity glucose sensor using a biocompatible glucose-responsive polymer. Sens Actuators B Chem. 2009 Jul 16;140(2): 603–609.

[14] Lueke J, Moussa WA. MEMS-based power generation techniques for implantable biosensing applications. Sensors (Basel). 2011;11(2):1433–60.

[15] Balaconis MK, Billingsley K, Dubach MJ, Cash KJ, Clark HA. The design and development of fluorescent nano-optodes for in vivo glucose monitoring. J Diabetes Sci Technol. 2011 Jan 1;5(1):68–75.

[16] Balaconis MK, Luo Y, Clark HA. Glucose-sensitive nanofiber scaffolds with an improved sensing design for physiological conditions. Analyst. 2015 Feb 7;140(3):716–23.

[17] Wu TY, Su YY, Shu WH, et al. A novel sensitive pathogen detection system based on Microbead Quantum Dot System. Biosens Bioelectron. 2016 Apr 15;78:37–44.

[18] Zhang H, Xu T, Li CW, Yang M. A microfluidic device with microbead array for sensitive virus detection and genotyping using quantum dots as fluorescence labels. Biosens Bioelectron. 2010 Jul 15;25(11):2402–7.

[19] Fu X, Cheng Z, Yu J, Choo P, Chen L, Choo J. A SERS-based lateral flow assay biosensor for highly sensitive detection of HIV-1 DNA. Biosens Bioelectron. 2016 Apr 15;78:530–7.

[20] Tsang MK, Ye W, Wang G, Li J, Yang M, Hao J. Ultrasensitive detection of Ebola virus oligonucleotide based on upconversion nanoprobe/nanoporous membrane system. ACS Nano. 2016 Jan 26;10(1):598–605.

[21] Mannoor MS, Zhang S, Link AJ, McAlpine MC. Electrical detection of pathogenic bacteria via immobilized antimicrobial peptides. Proc Natl Acad Sci USA. 2010 Nov 9;107(45):19207–12.

[22] Lillehoj PB, Kaplan CW, He J, Shi W, Ho CM. Rapid, electrical impedance detection of bacterial pathogens using immobilized antimicrobial peptides. J Lab Autom. 2014 Feb; 19(1):42–9.

[23] Cho IH, Irudayaraj J. In-situ immuno-gold nanoparticle network ELISA biosensors for pathogen detection. Int J Food Microbiol. 2013 Jun 3;164(1):70–5.

[24] Mevold AH, Hsu WW, Hardiansyah A, et al. Fabrication of gold nanoparticles/graphene-PDDA nanohybrids for bio-detection by SERS nanotechnology. Nanoscale Res Lett. 2015 Dec;10(1):397.

[25] Li S, Liu H, Deng Y, Lin L, He N. Development of a magnetic nanoparticles microarray for simultaneous and simple detection of foodborne pathogens. Biomed Nanotechnol. 2013 Jul;9(7):1254–60.

[26] Gao A1, Lu N, Dai P, Fan C, Wang Y, Li T. Direct ultrasensitive electrical detection of prostate cancer biomarkers with CMOS-compatible n- and p-type silicon nanowire sensor arrays. Nanoscale. 2014 Nov 7;6(21):13036–42.

[27] Mohd Azmi MA, Tehrani Z, Lewis RP, et al. Highly sensitive covalently functionalised integrated silicon nanowire biosensor devices for detection of cancer risk biomarker. Biosens Bioelectron. 2014 Feb 15;52:216–24.

[28] Chikkaveeraiah BV, Bhirde A, Malhotra R, Patel V, Gutkind JS, Rusling JF. Single-wall carbon nanotube forest arrays for immunoelectrochemical measurement of four protein biomarkers for prostate cancer. Anal Chem. 2009 Nov 1;81(21):9129–34.

[29] Takahashi S, Shiraishi T, Miles N, Trock BJ, Kulkarni P, Getzenberg RH. Nanowire analysis of cancer-testis antigens as biomarkers of aggressive prostate cancer. Urology. 2015 Mar;85(3):704.e1–7.

[30] Lee SK, Kim GS, Wu Y, et al. Nanowire substrate-based laser scanning cytometry for quantitation of circulating tumor cells. Nano Lett. 2012 Jun 13;12(6):2697–704.

[31] Shehada N, Brönstrup G, Funka K, Christiansen S, Leja M, Haick H. Ultrasensitive silicon nanowire for real-world gas sensing: noninvasive diagnosis of cancer from breath volatolome. Nano Lett. 2015 Feb 11;15(2):1288–95.

[32] Tran DP, Wolfrum B, Stockmann R, et al. Complementary metal oxide semiconductor compatible silicon nanowires-on-a-chip: fabrication and preclinical validation for the detection of a cancer prognostic protein marker in serum. Anal Chem. 2015 Feb 3;87(3):1662–8.

[33] Lu N, Gao A, Dai P, et al. CMOS-compatible silicon nanowire field-effect transistors for ultrasensitive and label-free microRNAs sensing. Small. 2014 May 28;10(10):2022–8.

[34] Huber F, Lang HP, Backmann N, Rimoldi D, Gerber C. Direct detection of a BRAF mutation in total RNA from melanoma cells using cantilever arrays. Nat Nanotechnol. 2013 Feb;8(2):125–9.

[35] Wang J, Wang S, Wang X, Zhu Y, Yang J. Cantilever array sensor for multiple liver cancer biomarkers detection. Sensors. 2014;2014:343–346.

[36] Liu Y, Li X, Zhang Z, Zuo G, Cheng Z, Yu H. Nanogram per milliliter-level immunologic detection of alpha-fetoprotein with integrated rotating-resonance microcantilevers for early-stage diagnosis of heptocellular carcinoma. Biomed Microdevices. 2009 Feb;11(1):183–91.

[37] Jokerst JV, Raamanathan A, Christodoulides N, et al. Nano-bio-chips for high performance multiplexed protein detection: determinations of cancer biomarkers in serum and saliva using quantum dot bioconjugate labels. Biosens Bioelectron. 2009 Aug 15;24(12):3622–9.

[38] Gazouli M, Lyberopoulou A, Pericleous P, et al. Development of a quantum-dot-labelled magnetic immunoassay method for circulating colorectal cancer cell detection. World J Gastroenterol. 2012 Aug 28;18(32):4419–26.

[39] Wang Y, Zhang Y, Du Z, Wu M, Zhang G. Detection of micrometastases in lung cancer with magnetic nanoparticles and quantum dots. Int J Nanomed. 2012;7:2315–24.

[40] Guo S, Chen YQ, Lu NN, Wang XY, Xie M, Sui WP. Ultrasonication-assisted one-step self-assembly preparation of biocompatible fluorescent-magnetic nanobeads for rare cancer cell detection. Nanotechnology. 2014 Dec 19;25(50):505603.

[41] Kanwar SS, Dunlay CJ, Simeone DM, Nagrath S. Microfluidic device (ExoChip) for on-chip isolation, quantification and characterization of circulating exosomes. Lab Chip. 2014 Jun 7;14(11):1891–900.

Chapter 7

Phage Display-Derived Antibodies: Application of Recombinant Antibodies for Diagnostics

Angela Chiew Wen Ch'ng, Yee Siew Choong and Theam Soon Lim

Additional information is available at the end of the chapter

http://dx.doi.org/10.5772/63927

Abstract

Antibodies are produced by the human body in response towards infections as a means of protection. The *in vivo* production of antibodies by B-cells involves a series of intricate gene editing processes resulting in a highly diverse pool of antibodies. However, this diversity can be replicated *in vitro* using phage display. Phage display offers the potential to present the antibody phenotype together with the cloned genotype of the specific antibody in a single-phage particle. Antibodies are highly sought after for diagnostic applications owing to its specificity and affinity towards a target antigen. The advent of recombinant antibody (rAb) technology allows for a faster and more cost-effective solution for antibody generation. It also provides diagnostic developers with the possibility to customize the antibodies. Antibodies have been utilized successfully in various diagnostic platforms ranging from standard immunoassays to lateral-flow assays, nanoparticles, microfluidics, DNA-integrated assays and others. The limitless application of antibodies in the field of diagnostics has made it a critical component in any diagnostic development platform. This chapter focuses on the processes involved in antibody discovery including the various forms of antibody libraries for phage display and panning processes. We also highlight some diagnostic platforms that apply recombinant antibodies.

Keywords: diagnostics, monoclonal antibodies, phage display, scFv, Fab, VHH

1. Introduction

The human body is made up of a series of complex networks or systems that involve different tissues and cells to work in harmony to regulate different functions in the human body. The immune system is one of the vital systems in the human body as its main function is to protect the body from infectious agents and pathogens. The immune system is divided into two main forms of immunity, namely the innate and acquired immunity. The innate immunity is the physical barrier that prevents foreign invasion. If the innate immunity fails to inhibit the entrance of these foreign molecules, the second line of defence being the adaptive immunity will then come into play. This response will take place with the help of both T- and B-cell [1]. B-cell activation to secrete antibodies can work through either the T-cell dependent or the T-cell independent pathway. The T-cell dependent activation would require T-helper cells to trigger the processes required for antibody production through B-cell proliferation [2]. This will then lead to the secretion of antibodies in the body.

Over decades, the application and function of antibodies has expanded from being an immunologically important protein to an essential research tool. The basic application of antibodies surrounds the natural feature of antibodies being high affinity and specific binders against target molecules. This feature has allowed antibodies to be successfully applied for diagnostic and therapeutic applications. In general, diagnostic kits are likely to apply antibodies with superior affinities and specificity against a target antigen for detection [3] via different orientations. This includes either the detection of antibodies by antigens, detection of serum antibodies by the corresponding antigens or by competition [4, 5].

Antibodies are a form of recognition protein [6], which is ubiquitously found in serum and body fluid of vertebrates. The diverse antibody repertoire is important for the identification of antibodies against a specific target. Antibodies undergo gene rearrangement processes to generate different gene segment combinations that result in antibodies with different gene sequences. The complexity of antibody diversity is mainly attributed to the combinatorial joining of multiple V, D, J segments of the heavy chain and the V, J segment for the light chain. This process involves multiple gene-editing enzymes to produce numerous combinations of gene segments. After gene segmentation, another process named somatic hypermutation takes place to further diversify the antibody repertoire [7, 8]. Taken together, these processes are mainly responsible for the highly diverse repertoire of antibodies found in the human body. This variation is the basis of the existence of different antigen-binding specificities and affinities of immunoglobulins (Igs) [2, 9].

The story of antibodies can be dated back to 1890, with the first report detailing the presence of antibodies and its function by Emil von Behring and Shibasaburo Kitasato. They used serum from animals immunized against diphtheria for administration to other animals infected with diphtheria and subsequently curing the infected animals [10, 11]. However, Paul Ehrlich in 1900 proposed the side-chain theory based on his hypothesis that the binding ability of a receptor is based on the side chains available for binding [12]. The side-chain theory was then supported by the 'lock and key' hypothesis by Emil Fischer that focused the hypothesis mainly on enzyme functions [12]. The constant evolution and understanding of immunology has helped open new avenues of antibody application and function.

Another major breakthrough in antibody technology development is the introduction of hybridoma technology. Traditionally, antibody production for diagnostic applications involved the use of animals. The immunization of animals with an immunogenic protein with and without an adjuvant would generally produce a collection of polyclonal antibodies [13]. A polyclonal pool of antibodies is defined as a set of heterogeneous antibodies targeting a specific antigen at multiple epitopes. The ability to identify monospecific antibodies only came about after Kohler and Milstein introduced the hybridoma technology in 1975. Hybridoma technology allows for monoclonal antibodies (MAbs) to be produced by fusing myeloma cells with antibody-producing spleen cells to create a hybrid exhibiting both characteristics [11]. This resulted in the formation of an immortal cell line with characteristics from both the spleenocytes and myeloma cells known as a hybridoma. The hybridomas are then screened until a single clone is obtained and the production of it is up-scaled. It is well known that antibodies generated via this manner are likely to have high affinities due to the maturation process that it underwent. Although successful, the process may be cumbersome and time consuming as researchers have found it at times difficult to generate antibodies using this method against toxic antigens, self-antigens and sensitive antigens such as membrane proteins or DNA. For all the benefits attributed to hybridoma technology, a major pitfall lies in the fact that for every new antigen a new animal host is required for immunization. Thus, it is difficult to predict or predefine the genetic information and epitope of the clone [11, 14]. This increases the difficulties, cost and time required to make antibodies, making it not the idle solution for antibody production [14].

This brought about a string of alternative methods for antibody production. The turn of the century saw the booming of molecular biology due to the success of recombinant DNA technology. Researchers were hard at work to develop the next alternative method for monoclonal antibody generation. This brought about various methods including phage display and other multiple display methods such as yeast display, ribosome display and mammalian cell display methods [14]. In addition, the use of transgenic animals was also introduced mainly with the xeno-mouse technology [11, 13, 14]. Even so, phage display is the preferred choice for recombinant antibody (rAb) production in most laboratories. Phage display allows for a faster and cost-effective solution towards antibody generation using Ff filamentous phage. In general, rAb production involves several steps including the generation of an antibody library, selection and enrichment of phage-displaying antibodies against specific antigens through the panning process, screening of monospecific antibodies and recombinant production of the antibodies via expression systems [15]. As phage-derived rAb may suffer from lower affinities, an additional stage of affinity maturation may be introduced to improve the antibodies produced. A major advantage to the use of phage display for rAb generation in contrast to conventional animal-derived methods is clearly the omission of animal use in the process. Another advantage of phage display is the lower downtime required for antibody production in between antigens. Conventional methods require immunization that may take up to weeks if not months to yield sufficient immune response for antibody production. This makes phage display rather efficient in the long term for antibody production process. However, one must acknowledge that phage-derived antibodies suffer from lower affinity when compared to conventional antibodies. This is due to the absence of affinity maturation in phage-derived antibodies as animal-derived antibodies are produced post maturation.

This chapter highlights monoclonal antibody development for diagnostic applications via phage display technology. This includes the different types of antibody libraries associated with antibody phage display. The chapter also highlights the different methods used to isolate antibodies against target antigens. The application of recombinant antibodies in different diagnostic platforms is also discussed briefly.

1.1. Phage display section

Phage display makes use of the natural replication cycle of bacteriophages to fuse a specific peptide or protein with the coat protein on the surface of the filamentous phage particles for selection. This design allows the presentation of a predefined foreign phenotype on the phage surface with the genotype being retrievable in the phage. This allowed a physical linkage between the phenotypic characteristics with the genotypic information to be established [11, 16–22].

There are two main methods for the display mechanism on phage. The first is with the use of a phage vector system, which allows the expression of coat protein III (pIII) to the foreign protein, in this case the antibodies are driven by the natural phage promoter [23, 24]. Additional helper phages are not required for phage packaging with phage vector systems. Unlike the phage vectors, the expression of the antibody-pIII protein by phagemid systems requires an artificial promoter such as the lac promoter. In addition, phagemid systems also require helper phage for phage packaging. As phagemid vectors do not carry the phage genome, complete phage packaging can only be done with the presence of the helper phage that carries the genetic information for the other proteins required for phage packaging. Therefore, a competition between wild-type pIII with the mutant pIII will occur. This difference in design of both phage and phagemid vectors also contributes to the display efficiency as phage systems are able to provide a multivalent display of the antibodies on pIII, whereas phagemid systems only allow monovalent display.

The isolation of antibody-presenting phages post binding with a target antigen allows simple identification of the clones by standard sequencing. Therefore, this approach has been utilized to introduce a collection of different antibody sequences into the phagemid vector to produce a collection of varying clones known as an antibody library [25]. The generation of antibody libraries will bring together a different set of considerations that is outlined in the following section.

2. Antibody library

For antibody isolation with phage display technology, a collection of antibodies has to be first made available. This involves the initial investment to generate a library of antibody clones to be presented on the surface of bacteriophages. The choice of library to be generated is rather dependent on its application, which would influence the subsequent decision-making process. This is because the type of library required would determine the source required and the minimum library size required ranging from 10^6 to 10^{10} [26]. In general, there are four main types of antibody libraries, namely naïve, immunized, synthetic and semi-synthetic library.

Naïve and synthetic antibodies are known as 'single-pot' libraries, which can be screened against any antigen [22, 26]. **Figure 1** shows the overall summary of all the libraries and their differences. However, each different library has its own particular characteristic that makes it preferred for certain applications. The application of phage display for antibody generation is not confined only to human antibodies but can also be applied to animal-derived antibodies.

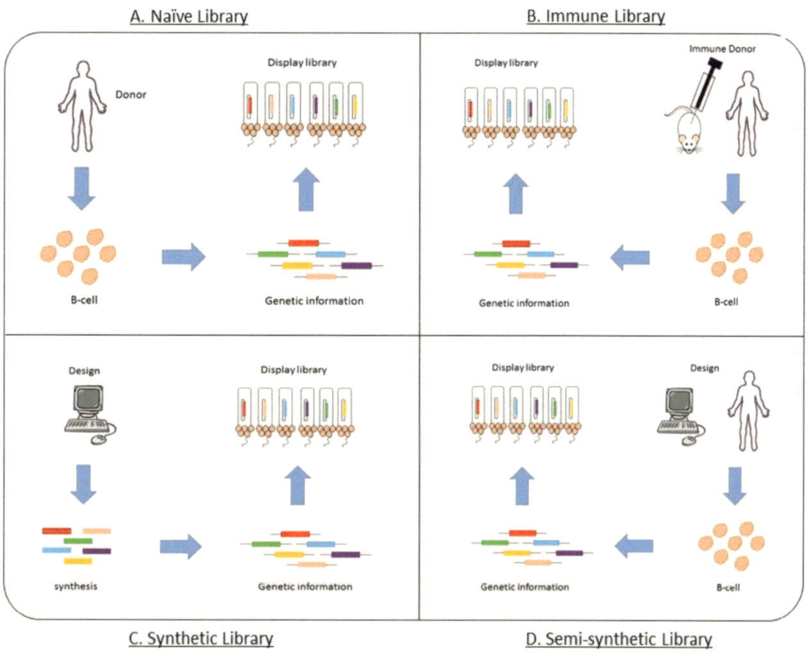

Figure 1. Types of antibody library design.

2.1. Naïve antibody library

Naïve antibody libraries are by definition a collection of antibody genes that are naïve in nature. In other words, the V-gene repertoire originates from IgM isotype of unimmunized or healthy donors [21]. The main characteristic of a naïve library is the unbiased nature of the repertoire. The antibody repertoire of healthy donors would mean no prior exposure or infection of the donors to any form of infection that could skew the immune response. As antibody production by the immune system is a direct response to the exposure of the individual to any pathogen, it is necessary for naïve libraries to obtain its repertoire from truly healthy donors.

The main advantage of a naïve or single-pot library is its large repertoire [22] for monoclonal antibody identification against numerous targets such as self, non-immunogenic or toxic substances. A technical bottleneck associated with naïve libraries is the sheer number of donors required as well as the number of theoretical diversity required. This would involve a large number of ligation and transformation experiments to achieve such numbers. A common problem of naïve libraries is the number of unknown and uncontrollable contents, such as the presence of memory cells of past infections that might influence the true nature of the naïve repertoire due to the huge naïve repertoire [27]. Another issue common to naïve libraries is the isolation of antibodies with varying degrees of affinities. It is common to obtain antibodies of modest affinities using naïve libraries, as the repertoire would have not undergone affinity maturation processes as opposed to hybridoma-derived or immunized library-derived antibodies.

The adaptation of naïve antibody libraries for diagnostic applications is not a new concept with several antibodies successfully being isolated for various diagnostic targets. Naïve libraries are useful for diagnostic as it can be used for selection against haptens, foreign and self-antigens. The ErBb2 protein, which is a tumour marker expressed by breast tumour, was selected against a naïve antibody library to obtain antibodies for immunoassay applications [28, 29]. **Table 1** summarizes the application of naïve antibody libraries to generate antibodies against a variety of antigens for diagnostic purpose.

Library	Library size	Source	Format	Target	Ref
Tu, 2016	2×10^7	Alpaca	sdAb (VHH)	*Listeria monocytogenes (LM)*	[27]
Yan, 2015	6.86×10^{11}	Camel	sdAbs	Human procalcitonin (PCT)	[28]
Ying, 2014	1×10^{12}	Human	Fabs	Receptor-binding domain of the MERS-CoV spike glycoprotein	[29]
Zhang, 2013	n/a	Human	Fabs	TES1 domain of the oncogenic LMP1	[30]
Boruah, 2013	n/a	Ilama	dsAbs	Glycoprotein of the Rabies virus (RABV)	[31]
Kirsch, 2008 (human naïve HAL4/7 antibody gene library)	5×10^9	Human	scFv	Alphavirus species (virus)	[32]
Velappan, 2007	n/a	Human	scFv	Sin Nombre Virus nucleocapsid protein (SNV-N)	[33]
Jiao, 2005	2×10^9	Human	Fabs	Receptor tyrosine kinase Met	[34]
McElhiney, 2000	1.47×10^8	Human	scFv	Microcystins	[35]
Sheets, 1998	6.7×10^9	Human	scFv	ErbB2 protein, Malaria (rPfHRP2)	[25, 36]

Table 1. Examples of naïve antibody libraries applied for diagnostic applications.

2.2. Synthetic and semi-synthetic antibody library

The antibody-binding region is located at the three complementarity-determining regions (CDRs) of the variable region in both the light chain and heavy chain. The gene sequences along the CDR are highly heterogeneous as a consequences of gene diversification such as V(D)J gene recombination, class switching and somatic hypermutation. The randomization in

http://dx.doi.org/10.5772/63927

the CDR is responsible for the varying affinities as well as specificity to all target antigens. DNA technology advancement encourages synthetic antibody design and synthesis at a reasonable cost in laboratory with the help of structural bioinformatics. This is because the prediction of antibody-antigen interaction can be done after considering the antibody structural constraints and preference.

It is with this information that antibody engineers are now able to design, improve and generate customized frameworks for antibody production. The ability to synthesize specific gene sequences and codons has made it possible to introduce randomization at the CDR. In general, CDR3 are found to be the region with the highest diversification other than CDR1 and CDR2 [30]. In addition to gene randomization, antibody-binding site was altered by inserting preferential amino acids that can also be used to introduce specific criteria to the antibody-binding sites. Another key factor is the CDR length that can also be predefined by the user.

In the context of synthetic antibody libraries, the natural immune maturation and somatic hypermutation process can be elevated to generate similar quality antibodies. To construct a synthetic library, the unarranged and randomized V-gene segments are synthetically assembled ex vivo normally by polymerase chain reaction (PCR). However, customization can be done on the genetic sequence, local variability and overall diversity for synthetic libraries unlike naïve libraries. Even specific codon usage can be applied to suit the needs of the user. Modifications to the framework can be carried out to improve features such as solubility and heat stability [31]. The main criterion for synthetic libraries to be beneficial is the theoretical diversity of the library. As the repertoire is largely naïve, the potential combinations generated by synthetic methods are able to rival the process carried out naturally with the large library size. However, the sheer size of the library diversity makes it difficult to re-culture without eventual loss of diversity. Even so, the antibodies enriched from synthetic libraries showed comparable affinities to those derived naturally [32]. Another major bottleneck associated with the use of synthetic libraries is the cost of generating a synthetic library. Even so, the turn of events in genetic engineering over the past few years has seen the cost for oligonucleotide synthesis reduced tremendously. Therefore, now it is a plausible solution for most laboratories to generate their own version of a synthetic antibody library.

A key subset of synthetic libraries is the production of semi-synthetic libraries. The first semi-synthetic library was reported in 1992, in which rearrangement of 49 human VH gene segments with five to eight residues of synthetic CDR was carried out to yield a semi-synthetic single-chain fragment variable (scFv) library [33]. The key difference between semi- and fully synthetic libraries is the source of the diversity. In semi-synthetic libraries, the diversity is largely obtained from natural sources whereby the genes encoding the CDR are isolated. These CDR genes are then inserted to a fixed framework sequence, which encodes the antibody backbone [27, 34]. The diversity is still natural, taking advantage of the maturation processes of antibodies *in vivo*. The application of synthetic antibodies to develop antibodies for diagnostic applications has allowed the generation of antibodies against various antigens of diagnostic value.

This is evident with approximately three billion clones in the ETH-2-Gold library that were used against a wide range of recombinant antigens, such as extracellular glycoprotein of tenascin-C (TNC) [35]. Other versions have been reported such as the Tomlinson I library with 18 amino acid side-chain diversity on the CDR, and the Griffin library [36] was constructed by using six diverse synthetic CDR3 regions [37]. The main difference between Tomlinson I and J libraries is the choice of randomization used before clone into pIT2 phagemid system. The Tomlinson I library uses the DVT degeneracy to introduce diversity at the CDR. The Tomlinson J library makes use of the NNK degeneracy in the CDR design. Nucleotide degeneracy is commonly used to introduce mutations in the codon at the CDR regions that are responsible for antigen-binding specificity and affinity. DVT and NNK degeneracy are generic codons abiding a specific formula for base usage. The base usage of each degeneracy is as follows: D is 33% G/33% A/33% T; V is 33% G/33% A/33% C; N is any nucleic acid and K is 50% G/50% T. When the degeneracy is translated as a codon, it will yield multiple combinations of amino acids to increase the diversity of the gene. The application of different degenerate codons also allows the application of different groups of amino acids in the CDR design. The antibodies isolated from these libraries could then be used as a diagnostic tool [37, 38].

The HuCAL library from Morphosys is a famous fully synthetic antibody library with predefined randomized frameworks [39]. The different versions of the HuCAL libraries, namely HuCAL Gold and HuCAL Platinum, were generated with six trinucleotide-randomized CDRs [40, 41], whereas HuCAL and HuCAL Gold libraries were made with seven VH, four VK and three Vλ germline families. This allows the generation of 49 framework combination of the VH-VL [42]. Structural diversity of the CDR was introduced by randomization of CDR1, CDR2 and CDR3 [39]. Another version of the HuCAL library is the HuCAL Platinum that consists of seven VH, three VK and three Vλ framework sequences. HuCAL Platinum was designed without the use of VH4 and VK4 as they are found to be rare [43]. The HuCAL libraries have been used also for antibody generation for the diagnosis of bovine insulin [39, 40, 42]. **Table 2** shows a list of some known fully-synthetic and semi-synthetic libraries used for diagnostic applications.

Library	Type	Diversity generation	Format	Target	Ref
Synthetic phage display nanobody (Nb) library	Synthetic	Degenerate codon NNK	scAbs (VHH)	Human prealbumin (PA) and neutrophil gelatinase-associated lipocalin (NGAL)	[50]
Synthetic	Synthetic	–	scFv	Coronary artery disease (CAD)	[51]
ETH-2-Gold library	Synthetic	–	scFv	Extracellular glycoprotein C-domain of tenascin-C (TNC)	[42]
Ylanthia Library	Synthetic	Fixed VH/VL framework pairs selected on biophysical characteristics	Fab	Recombinant human (rh) ErbB4, rhFZD4/Fc, rhTNFalpha, M-CSF, eGFP	[49, 52]

Library	Type	Diversity generation	Format	Target	Ref
HuCAL Gold	Synthetic	7 VH, 4 VK and 3 Vλ germline family	scFv, Fab	IL18R-Fc, -Gal, Est-BSA	[46, 48]
HuCAL Platinum	Synthetic	7 VH, 3 VK and 3 Vλ framework	Fab	Human TRAIL R2/Fc and rhIL-2Rαalpha;/Fc fusion protein	[47]
Tomlinson I Library	Synthetic	DVT side chain	scFv	Microcystins, ferritin, SARS-associated corona virus	[35, 51, 53]
Griffin Library	Semi-synthetic	–	scFv	Microcystins	[43, 44]
Tomlinson J Library	Semi-synthetic	NNK side chain	scFv	SARS-associated corona virus	[53]

Table 2. A list of fully-synthetic and semi-synthetic libraries and application in diagnostics.

2.3. Immunized library

The immunized library repertoire originates from V-gene of immunized donors [27] or disease-infected donors. In immunized libraries, the immunized repertoire would be specific for one antigen or a collection of antigens specific for a particular disease. This limits the use of the libraries when compared to naïve and synthetic libraries. Even so, the V-genes are collected from donors that have been exposed to the target antigen allowing isolation of higher-affinity antibodies using such libraries. These antibody libraries mainly produce antibodies of good affinities with high clonal diversity due to *in vivo* somatic hypermutation that contributes towards affinity maturation. This would influence the library diversity in a way that the final library size required does not necessarily need to be as high as naïve libraries [26]. This is useful to study disease immune responses, vaccination strategies and human immunity. The major setback to such libraries is the need to generate a new library to study every different disease [22, 26, 27].

Several different libraries have been developed for various diseases such as hepatitis B [44] and those listed in **Table 3**. These libraries contain a plethora of useful antibodies that are specific to the disease making it a valuable asset for infectious diseases. The generation of immunized libraries is not restricted to humans but can also be carried out in animals such as mice. Immunization of mice with the target antigen would likely yield a library of clones against the specific target protein. Although this may not differ much from the conventional hybridoma technology, however, conversion to a recombinant version would allow easy up-scaling for production and also for modification.

Library	Source	Format	Target for diagnosis	Ref
Gong, 2015	Camel	sdAbs (VHH)	H7N2 virus	[61]
Prantner, 2015	Human	sdAbs	Mesothelin cancer biomarker	[62]
Zhou, 2015	Chicken	scFv	Bursal disease virus (VP2 protein)	[63]

Library	Source	Format	Target for diagnosis	Ref
Hosking, 2015	Buffalo	scFv	Schistosome infection	[64]
Zhou, 2015	Rainbow trout	scFv	Viral haemorrhagic septicaemia, VHS (viral haemorrhagic septicaemia virus, VHSV)	[65]
Unger, 2015	Ilamas/camelid	scAbs (VHH)	*Clostridium difficile* toxin (CDT)	[66]
Li, 2015	Camel	scAbs (VHH)	Coronary artery disease, CAD (Apolipoprotein B-100)	[67]
Sabir, 2014	Camel	sdAbs (VHH)	Tuberculosis (TB)	[68]
Shahi, 2014	Camel	scAbs (VHH)	Botulinum neurotoxin E (BoNT/E)	[69]
Mohammadzadeh, 2014	Mice	scFv	HIV-1 capsid protein p24	[70]
Li, 2014	Chicken	scFv	Newcastle disease virus (NDV)	[71]
Yang, 2014	Camel	scAbs (VHH)	Porcine circovirus type 2 (PCV2)	[72]
Zhu, 2014	Camel	scAbs (VHH)	Influenza H3N2	[73]
Chiliza, 2008	Chicken	scFv	Malaria	[74]
Cumming, 1998	Mice	scFv	*Mycobacterium tuberculosis* (65-kDa Mtb antigen)	[75]

Table 3. A list of immunized antibody libraries and application in diagnostics.

Immunized libraries have been used successfully in developing antibodies against diagnostic biomarkers. This can be seen with the application of this concept for epitopes of immunogenic antigen, such as carcinoembryonic antigen (CEA) [32, 45]. Anti-CEA antibodies can be applied for targeting and to image colorectal tumours. This transcends the conventional diagnostic platforms allowing *in vivo* cell staining or even with clinical imaging technologies. Besides, immune Fab antibody libraries were used to isolate antibody clones against human immunodeficiency virus type 1 (HIV-1), respiratory syncytial virus (RSV) and herpes simplex virus (HSV) [46]. Additionally, hepatitis A antibodies were isolated from hepatitis A immune library against CR236 via serodiagnostic immune adherence test (IA) or complement-fixation (CF) test [47]. Diagnosis of heparin-induced immune thrombocytopenia (HIT) was made possible by using HIT antibodies from immune libraries. This is crucial as patients who have been diagnosed with HIT are required to stop heparin and start using alternate anticoagulant for treatment [48, 49]. Diagnosis of anthrax was done via detection against antigen *Bacillus anthracis* spores with immunized scFv antibody phage display library [50].

3. Selection and screening of antibody libraries

Panning is an *in vitro* selection method that functions to isolate antibody fragments based on their affinity towards the antigen from a diverse collection of clones. This approach is common for antibody development for diagnostics and therapeutic application [51, 52]. Before selection of antibodies can be carried out, the antibody libraries must be developed first. The constructed library must then be packaged as fusion protein on bacteriophage particles. The basic

http://dx.doi.org/10.5772/63927

principle involves accessibility of phage-presenting antibodies to bind to a target antigen based on affinity.

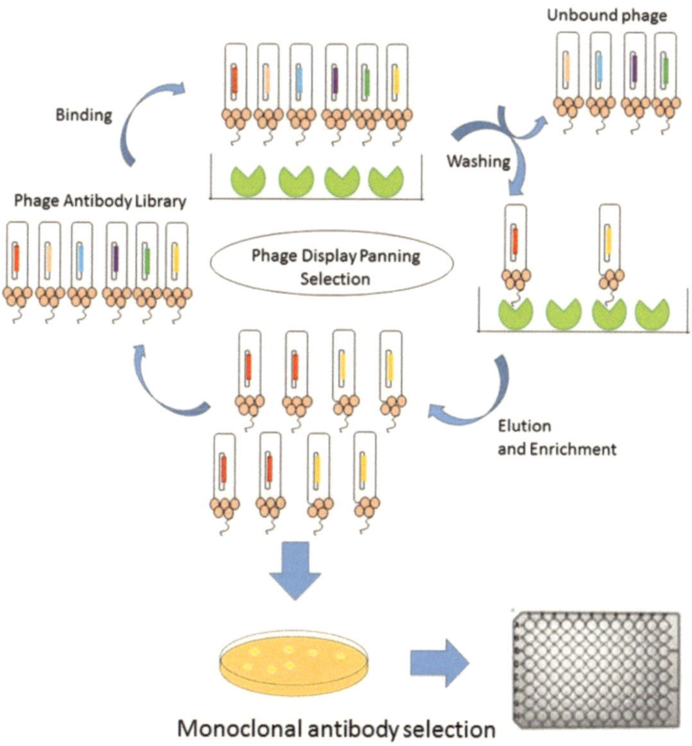

Figure 2. Antibody selection bio-panning protocol.

In this respect, (**Figure 2**) shows that the target antigen must first be immobilized on solid surfaces such as nitrocellulose, magnetic beads, column matrices or plastic surfaces in the form of polystyrene tube or 96-well microtitre plates [22]. In fact, the major difference among all the panning selection strategies is the immobilization surface where antigens are coated on. Other than this, parameters such as washing, elution and enrichment steps can be optimized for a successful selection process. As for evaluation, polyclonal and monoclonal antibody phage enzyme-linked immunosorbent assay (ELISA) is usually used to determine the presence of a positive clone after panning [53].

3.1. Conventional panning strategy

To date, there have been a number of different panning strategies reported for the isolation of MAbs against various antigens. Traditionally, the favoured method for most researchers is to immobilize or coat antigens on solid supports such as polystyrene immunotube and polystyrene immunoplate [53].

The attachment of antigen to the polystyrene surface can either be direct using surface-treated plates or by using intermediate capture mechanisms. This includes streptavidin-coated plates to capture biotinylated ligands (protein or peptide). The biotin-streptavidin mechanism is useful to avoid epitope disconformation during antigen immobilization on a plastic surface [54]. After the immobilization of antigen, phage-displayed libraries are incubated with the bound antigens for affinity capture. This was then continued with the washing of unbound phages before phage elution for rescue. Then, the eluted phage was subjected to amplification and precipitation steps for the following panning round until a positive clone is obtained [55]. Here, the wash step can be modified to introduce different degrees of stringency to specify certain characteristics required for the antibodies. This way, customization of the strategy helps to determine the final output characteristics.

3.2. High-throughput panning strategies

To increase the screening effectiveness, streptavidin magnetic beads can be used to coat the biotinylated antigens. A major advantage in using nanoparticles is the higher surface area to volume ratio for the capture of higher amount of targets. Magnetic-based panning allows multiple antigen screening at the same time. A semi-automated panning process includes manipulation of magnetic beads by multi-pin method, robotic arm or a robotic system during the panning process to increase the panning efficiency [56]. The main concept of panning using the semi-automated process applies a similar concept of affinity-based selection as the conventional method. The incubation, wash and elution steps are carried out with automation to improve reproducibility and accuracy. However, the phage rescue process is still carried out offline by manual infection. Even so, the process still utilizes significant automation to lower labour involvement and allows for high-throughput screening to be carried out.

The concept of full automation refers to a pipeline process without the involvement of any human, whereas semi-automation requires human involvement at some point of the process [53]. The main benefit that high-throughput panning brings to the process is a higher efficiency in selection with minimum labour as all the parameters can be easily programmed for repetitive steps. This also increases reproducibility of the incubation time, temperature, washing and elution condition. This allows for easy handling of multiple targets at the same time. Such protocols can help to reduce from 2 days to a single day for one selection cycle, which means only a week is required for the entire panning process. This method is easily automated with the use of magnetic particle processors such as the Kingfisher Flex system [56].

The next-generation phage display allows differentiation of unselected and selected phage after enrichment rounds [57] against a target antigen for both large combinatorial peptide and antibody libraries through DNA sequence analysis of the phenotype-bearing phage [51]. There are some similarities of this platform with conventional phage panning, where both includes laborious colony picking and functional ligand screening. The sheer number of clones to be analysed is easily overcome by the use of next-generation sequencers (NGSs). This strategy is cost-effective, fast and less labour intensive as compared to conventional phage display selection. Moreover, this technology improves the overall accuracy for large quantification. In terms of coverage, DNA deep sequencing through NGS offers a high coverage for full

http://dx.doi.org/10.5772/63927

repertoire of ligand particles. In short, high-throughput DNA sequencing through NGS method is cost-effective, provides higher accuracy and high coverage for large quantification especially for library screening [57].

Another method utilizing the mass spectrometry immunoassay (MSIA™) system was introduced where the separation of antibodies and antigen for mass spectrometry (MS) analysis is done via affinity. Previously, the MSIA™ method is an immune affinity method used in protein analyte purification for MS detection purposes. The MSIA™ tip was successfully used as a solid phase to carry out semi-automated panning for antibody enrichment. The MSIA™ tips that contain streptavidin that are covalently linked to a porous monolithic solid support will function as the capture molecule. The streptavidin capture molecules are best known for the easy capture of biotinylated target through biotin-streptavidin interaction. The MSIA™ tip method only requires the use of a standard electronic multichannel pipettor and an adjustable pipette stand. This method is also cost-effective for phage display panning as it does not require investments on instrumentation. However, the method can also be incorporated to larger pipetting instruments for antibody panning also. The panning protocol uses the similar concepts as conventional panning that includes incubation, washing and final elution. Then, bound phages are then amplified and used in the following panning rounds to obtain clonal enrichment. This method was reported to successfully identify antibodies against the hemolysin E antigen of *Salmonella typhi* [58]. In short, this method is also an attractive alternative for high-throughput screening.

3.3. Cell panning

Cell panning is an innovative screening method using whole fixed or live cells, tissue section or live animals expressing the antigen of interest for panning [22]. In other words, whole live cells serve as an antigen carrier to screen phage antibodies [59, 60]. All the selection methods mentioned were panned against purified antigens, but whole cell antigen is used in whole cell panning. This panning strategy is usually an alternative method for complex and difficult antigens which cannot be purified with similar properties, for example, cell surface receptor or antigen [60] is only functional when retained in lipid bilayers [59]. There are several parameters to consider when carrying out cell panning such as (1) quality of antibody library, (2) display manner, (3) antigen concentration and (4) cell-surface antigen density. This is to ensure the success of the panning process.

4. Antibody formats

Antibodies are normally identified in a Y-shape configuration. The variability is mainly due to the V-region (two arms of Y-end) as this is where the antigens bind [61]. Thus, smaller versions of antibody formats have been developed to take advantage of the binding specificities of the V-region. Due to advancement in recombinant DNA technology, a number of new antibody formats such as domain antibodies, single-chain fragment variable, tandem scFv, diabody, tetrabody, minibody and single-chain fragment antigen binding (scFab) have been introduced (**Figure 3**).

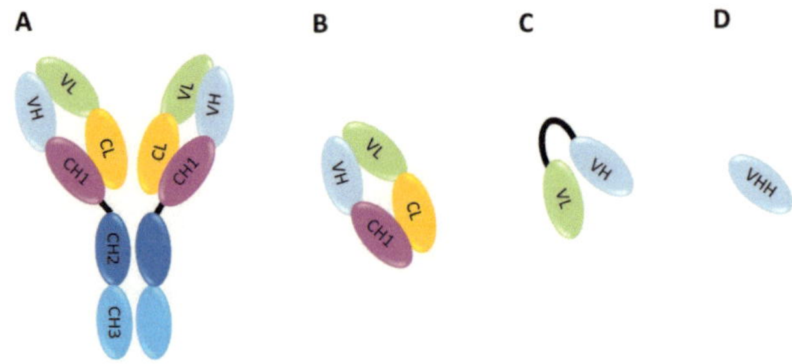

Figure 3. Antibody fragment design. (A) Full antibody; (B) fragment antibody binding (Fab); (C) single-chain fragment variable (scFv); and (D) single-domain antibody (sdAbs).

A main consideration of antibody formats is the size; smaller fragments have an advantage that they are able to retain the antigen-binding specificity and can be produced economically [26, 62]. This is important for application in diagnostics, as this will in turn contribute to lowering the production cost during manufacturing. The main consideration for any antibody to be used on a diagnostic platform is mainly the specificity and affinity of the antibody against the target antigen. These two characteristics are not lost with the use of smaller fragments albeit there will be no avidity effect with the monomeric smaller fragments.

Both scFv and Fab formats are commonly used in research and industrial applications, and are the preferred formats for presentation on phage [16, 20, 34, 62, 63]. This is because the expression of complete IgG is not suitable for *Escherichia coli* as the large size and post-translational modifications available are not designed for bacteria [64]. In the context of antibody formats for application in phage display, the smaller-sized formats are preferred due to the ease of expression and presentation efficiency. Larger native structures may not be tolerated well by the bacterial host required for the packaging of new phage particles. The following section will mainly discuss the antibody formats commonly used in phage display. This includes the domain antibodies, single-chain fragment variable and fragment antigen binding, which are truncated versions of the full immunoglobulin.

4.1. Domain antibody (dAb)

Domain antibodies are small (11–15 kDa) and consist only of either the VH or the VL domain [34]. Thus, they will only have three out of a possible six CDR from a full variable region consisting of both VH and VL. It was found that single-domain antibodies (sdAbs) are able to provide better stability as well as solubility when specific families such as the VH3 framework are used. The stability of the human VH domain antibody can be further enhanced by extending the length of CDRH3 loop [65], much like the hypervariable region of camelid VHH that are longer than the human VH. According to Ponsel and Neugebauer [34], camelid and cartilage fish's single-domain antibodies are more stable, with a high resistance towards aggregation and temperature due to the framework sequence [34, 66].

Domain antibodies can also penetrate tissue efficiently as compared to full-length IgG due to their smaller size. VHHs are commonly used as detection units on biosensor or immune-adsorbent to identify the presence of lysozyme, carbonic anhydrase, alpha-amylase [67], beta-lactamase or even act as a cancer-imaging agent. It was also used to detect the surface antigen of different hepatitis serotypes [66]. In addition, single-domain antibody is used due to an easier production system when compared to conventional antibodies because of the size and folding [56, 68]. As domain antibodies are devoid of any quaternary structure, production and stability of domain antibodies allows it to be used at extreme conditions. This provides great benefit for diagnostics, as the improved heat stability would allow easy transportation of antibodies without cold chain. This is especially beneficial for diagnostic kit development for in-field diagnosis of infectious diseases in areas with limited resources.

4.2. Single-chain antibody variable fragments of ~27 kDa

Single-chain antibody variable fragment is made up of VL and VH domain with a glycine-serine flexible linker in between to hold the domain in proximity to form the binding cavity upon folding [3]. In addition, GS linkers are known to improve the folding, flexibility and stability of the single-chain fragment variable as compared to proline-rich linker. This is because pro-rich sequence exhibits rigid and stiff conformation due to the absence of hydrogen at the amine, which forms hydrogen bonds with other amino acids [69]. Therefore, the scFv fragments are designed with six CDRs, thus increasing the diversity and repertoire of the antibodies. The scFv has been shown to bind to a variety of antigens, such as hapten, protein, carbohydrate, receptor, tumour antigen and viruses [63]. Moreover, small scFvs are easily folded and producible in *E. coli* for diagnostic applications too [3, 63, 64, 70].

As a linker joins the VH and VL domain physically, the single polypeptide composition helps to facilitate the production and folding in *E. coli* that allows for efficient presentation of antibody repertoire on phage surface [70, 71] due to better expression in *E. coli* [14, 71]. Thus, many libraries generated use the scFv fragment as the preferred format for selection [64, 72]. The scFv format has been used in whole blood agglutination assay for rapid diagnostic test for HIV-1 [71]. The scFv fragment was detected by tags in ELISA besides fusing with reporter enzyme to act as secondary antibody [73].

4.3. Fragment antibody-binding fragments of ~57 kDa

As a comparison to scFv, Fab fragments are composed of the VH, CH1 and entire VL fragment held together by interchain disulphide bonds. The Fab fragments have a tendency to form dimers which could cause problems with binding and affinity as it exerts the avidity effect [13]. *In vitro,* Fab expression vector is more complex than the scFv system as it consists of two separate polypeptide chains linked by the formation of a disulphide bridge. Thus, it is important to ensure a balanced expression of both antibody chains in order to allow good presentation of Fab on phage.

There are several designs used for Fab presentation that includes either the monocistronic or the bicistronic arrangement of antibody. The gene arrangement of a Fab fragment for phage display requires fusion of either VL or VH to the phage pIII coat protein. The production of the accompanying chain will be carried out simultaneously as an independent protein allowing it to locate each other at the periplasmic cavity to form disulphide bonds between them for proper presentation. This challenge is overcome by alternative approaches using molecular chaperones to improve the presentation of full Fab fragments during phage display and protein expression [74].

In diagnostic applications, Fab-peptide epitope and Fab-Fab bifunctional reagent were used to detect the HIV-1, HIV-2 and hepatitis B surface antigen, which were known as antibody-based reagent [71] in agglutination assays. **Table 4** shows the broad application of different antibody formats for diagnostic applications. There is no actual best format for diagnostics but is mainly subjected to the preference of the users and the diagnostic platform set-up.

Antibody fragment format	Source	Antigen	Disease	Ref
Single Domain antibody (sdAb)	Camel	Prostate-specific antigen (PSA)	Prostate cancer	[98]
	Semi-synthetic	*Mycobacterium tuberculosis* (MTb) α-crystalline	*Mycobacterium tuberculosis*	[99]
	Ilama	Marburg virus variants	Haemorrhagic fever	[100]
	Human	Protein C3a, cancer antigen, carcinoembryonic antigen, MUC family glycoproteins, autoantibodies, sialyl-LewisX and cytokines	Breast cancer	[101]
	Alpaca (VHH)	*Listeria monocytogens (LM)*	Food-borne pathogens	[27]
	Camel (VHH)	H7N2 virus	Avian influenza virus subtype H7N2	[61]
Single-chain fragment antibody (scFv)	Mice	*Bacillus anthracis* spores (exosporium)	Anthrax	[60]
	–	Domoic acid	Amnesic shellfish poisoning (ASP)	[102]
	Mouse	*Clostridium difficile* toxin B	*C. difficile* infection, cause of nosocomial diarrhoea	[103]
	Mice	Prostate-specific membrane antigen (PSMA)	Prostate cancer	[104]
Fragment antibody binding (Fab)	Human	Anti-carcinoembryonic antigen (CEA)	Colorectal carcinoma	[105]
	Mouse	prostate-specific antigen (PSA)	Prostate cancer	[106]
	Human	Hepatitis B surface antigen (HBsAg)	Hepatitis B	[54]

Table 4. Application of antibody fragment as diagnostic probe.

5. Application of recombinant antibodies in rapid diagnostics

Recombinant antibodies are used in diagnostics due to its binding specificity and affinity. There are many platforms, such as lateral-flow assay (LFA), ELISA and cell imaging available in the market today, which are rapid and accurate in identifying the target antigens found in sample. Most of the platforms make use of either the antigen-capture assay or the antibody-capture assay to diagnose the presence of certain diseases [75].

5.1. Lateral-flow dipstick assay

Lateral-flow assay or immunochromatography assays are normally found as a test strips with the most common being the pregnancy test strip. The theory behind lateral-flow assay is based on the capillary action that occurs in the nitrocellulose membrane to migrate molecules along the membrane to cause a reaction and detect target antigen [75, 76]. This is because the presence of antigens in the sample matrix against a specific antibody reflects the onset of certain disease and treatment should be carried out immediately. (**Figure 4**) shows the actual design, polyclona antibodies against the target antigen were conjugated with gold nanoparticles and are deposited on the membrane. The migration of the sample when mixed with the antibody-coated particles will allow the particles to flow along the membrane until it is captured by a secondary antibody that is permanently fixed along the membrane as a line. Therefore, the presence of the antigen will be reported by the appearance of a band on the dipstick that represents the concentration of the gold nanoparticles on the target line.

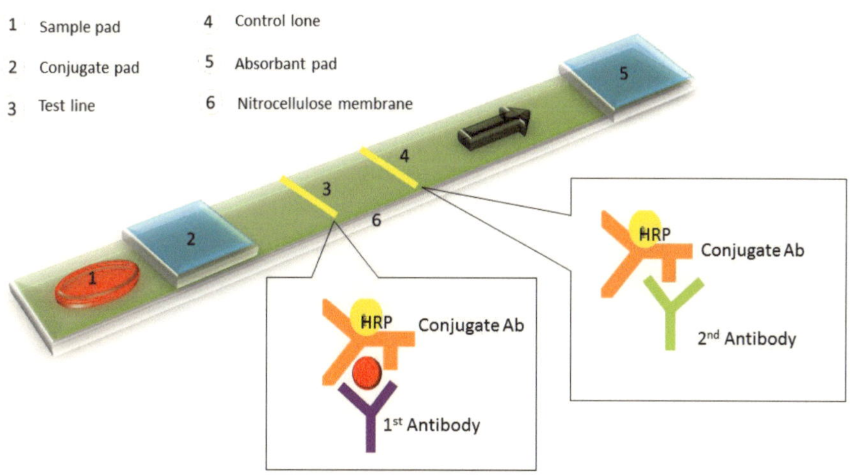

Figure 4. Lateral-flow dipstick assay design.

The conventional design of the lateral-flow strips will show a single control line and another test line. The control line indicates the control assay to show that the lateral-flow system is in order. The working assay requires buffer to improve the performance as well as the compatibility with other components used in assay. There are two formats used in LFAs, sandwich and competitive format [77]. In short, dipstick assay is sensitive enough to detect the antigen constituent within 10 min besides the simple usage that does not require professional personnel to carry out the test. The conjugation of recombinant antibodies to gold nanoparticles is essential for the generation of lateral-flow assays. The ability to produce recombinant antibodies easily using bacterial expression systems would facilitate rapid kit production at a lower cost.

5.2. Microfluidic platform

Microfluidics makes use of the movement of small amounts of fluid along a small diameter channel. Microfluidics was vastly applied due to the small sample volume needed for fast and precise result. The microfluidic platform is highly sensitive, efficient and portable [78].

Recent developments in microfluidic technology including on-chip detection and imaging, on-chip flow cytometry, on-chip immunoassay and nanosensor for point of care (POC) diagnostic application [79] help to overcome conventional ELISA's limitation for immunoassay-based diagnosis; micro-ELISA systems have been proposed for sensitive and rapid diagnostics using a fluidic chamber. This modified ELISA platform uses a microfluidic platform that reduces the amount of sample required by 10 times (<10 μL), 20 times faster analysis (<20 min) with a higher sensitivity range (Um–pM) as compared to conventional ELISA [79, 80]. Rapid diagnosis is the most important selling point for biomarkers such as protein, carbohydrate, lipid, metabolites, genomic DNA and RNA by using immunoassay due to the obvious advantage in disease management.

To improve the quantitative result, fluid-handling components and data acquisition software were used. In addition, microfluidic kits are integrated with electrical, optical and mechanical transducer to improve the platform [79, 80]. Other than that, the development of on-chip diffusion assay allows the measurement of small molecules within the microfluidic channels. This is done by detection of the labelled probe by antibodies against the probe itself. This study also proves that microfluidic diffusion is suitable for blood sample analysis [81]. There have been other versions of assays utilizing recombinant antibodies in fluidic platforms such as malaria detection with on-card dry reagent storage of microfluidic immunoassay from blood samples [79].

5.3. Enzyme-linked immunosorbent assay

The ELISA platform takes advantage of the specific interaction between antibody and antigens to allow a capture base for detection. The method requires a series of incubation and wash steps, which can be time consuming and tedious. Thus, antigens are first coated on a microtitre plate and then blocked overnight before incubation with antibodies. To detect binding between antigen and antibody, bio-conjugate and chemical-conjugate proteins coupled with reporter enzymes such as horseradish peroxidase (HRP) or alkaline phosphatase (AP) are used. Lastly, 2,2′-azino-bis(3-ethylbenzothiazoline-6-sulphonic acid) (ABTS) is used as a colour indicator for successful binding between antigen and antibody. However, the conventional ELISA approach has setbacks such as long assay time, large amount of expensive antibodies, chemicals, plastic ware and liquid-handling platforms. This process although straightforward may still require professional training in order to minimize any false-positive result and ensure reproducibility [82].

5.4. Nanoparticles, silica, polystyrene and latex agglutination test (LAT)

The advent of nanotechnology has brought about the introduction of nanosized particles and with it a series of new diagnostic platforms. There are many nanoparticles that have been used for diagnostic platforms. This includes gold nanoparticles (AuNPs) [83–86], carbon nanotubes and carbon nanoparticles (CNPs) [87]. The chemical property of these nanoparticles has allowed the expansion of the diagnostic platforms from simple colorimetric assays to the introduction of electrical signal, fluorescence and even phase transition readouts [83–85].

Although the use of AuNPs is associated with its application in lateral-flow dipstick assay as the immobilization surface for DNA, antibodies and proteins for the line development, it has also been used independent of the lateral flow. An assay was developed using AuNPs with influenza-specific antibodies acting as labels to detect influenza virus. This will result in the AuNPs probe aggregating and causing a readout in dynamic light-scattering (DLS) spectroscopy. Thus, the detection of AuNP aggregation was analysed using the DLS to determine the concentration of virus present. This method monitors the size change of aggregated nanoparticles and not change colour. However, the DLS approach is more suitable in detecting larger viruses with multiple epitopes [88].

The latex antigen detection or latex immunoagglutination test established in 1959 makes use of protein-conjugated latex microspheres to magnify the antigen-antibody interaction [89]. This LAT assay is fast and simple to use for the diagnosis of circulating antigens in patients with systemic infection because latex is sensitized with the serum of an immune donor [90]. The latex complexes will agglutinate if the target antigen is present [91]. The LAT platform has been used for the diagnosis of systemic candidiasis [90, 91], visceral leishmaniasis [89], invasive pulmonary aspergillosis [92], *Helicobacter pylori* infection [93] and *Meningococcal meningitis* [94]. The diagnostic test can be done using blood, cerebrospinal fluid or other body fluids depending on the design of the agglutination test.

5.5. Fusion with DNA technology—DNAzyme probe system, immuno-PCR (IPCR), immuno-quadruplex priming amplification (IQPA), immuno-rolling circle amplification (IRCA)

Enzyme-linked immunosorbent assay is an assay that uses the enzymatic reaction as a basis of reporting. However, such assays sometimes suffer from a lack of sensitivity to detect low-dose drugs or biomarkers [95]. To overcome this issue, the fusion of DNA technology with protein engineering has brought about newer reporter systems that can increase the sensitivity of assays. This includes modified hybrid methods such as antigen-DNAzyme, immuno-PCR, immuno-QPA and immuno-RCA.

The antigen-DNAzyme-based probe reporter system is a simple and rapid immuno-based assay that depends on the peroxidase activity as a reporter signal and the affinity of antigen-antibody for binding. DNAzymes also known as deoxyribozyme, founded by Ronald Breaker and Gerald Joyce in the year 1994, are catalytically active DNA molecules, which are able to function mimicking enzymatic reactions [96]. G-quadruplex (G-quad) structures are formed by guanine-rich nucleic acids. The guanine-rich sequence will form a guanine tetrad structure with intra-Hoogsteen hydrogen bonding. This will then allow two or more guanine tetrads bind to form a G-quad. The G-quad structure is further stabilized by the presence of cations. The complexation of G-quad structures with a hemin will form a peroxidase mimicking DNAzyme that catalyses the peroxidase-mediated oxidation of ABTS [97, 98]. The main difference of this antibody-antigen detection assay is the use of G-quad DNA structures in association with hemin as a reporter system. The addition of hemin to a G-quad structure will allow the transfer of electrons from the guanine to hemin in the presence of peroxide to oxidize the ABTS to form a green complex that is visible to the eye [98].

This assay design allows the fusion of the G-quad to function as a DNAzyme to generate a colorimetric readout as a reporter system for the rapid detection of small haptens such as hormones or drug molecules [99]. Thus, DNAzyme can be conjugated with antibodies for signal enhancement with the help of hemin and is suitable to be used as an immunoassay in biodiagnostic platforms [98]. As the G-quad sequence is made up of oligonucleotides, the sensitivity of the assay can be greatly improved via external DNA amplification processes to generate more G-quad sequences for reaction with hemin.

Immuno-quadruplex priming amplification is another hybrid method that couples both the calorimetric DNAzyme detection with an effective DNA amplification for improved sensitivity. IQPA is an immunoassay platform that generates G-quad reporter molecules via an isothermal quadruplex-priming amplification process. The reporter G-quad forming sequences, which were amplified from isothermal QPA, allow QPA to fuse with an immunoassay platform. In other words, we can avoid reporter conjugate enzyme in the immunoassay platform. QPA employs a set of primer and enzyme to maintain the stringent condition for target amplification to generate multiple copies of the G-quad sequence at an isothermal condition. Streptavidin can be sandwiched between the antigen and antibody DNA to form the binding for IQPA to work. The hemin molecules are then used complex with the amplified G-quad structures to catalyse the colour change of ABTS in the presence of hydrogen peroxide [100].

Immuno-PCR is another hybrid immuno-based assay that combines ELISA-type ligand-binding assay (LBA) technologies with PCR amplification signal without the use of antibody-enzyme conjugates. As a replacement, antibody-DNA conjugates were used whereby the DNA marker is physically linked to the capture antibody and a polymerase chain reaction step is introduced to generate copies of the DNA sequence. This allows improvements of 100–10,000-fold in limit of detection (LOD) as compared to conventional ELISA [95, 101]. Although the LOD of IPCR is almost in line with the ligand-binding assay, IPCR assay has been considered as challenging. Thus, various modifications are required to increase its sensitivity. This includes technical issues such as the availability of thermostable enzymes, high protein-binding capacity microplates and minimizing cross-contamination by avoiding plate trans-

http://dx.doi.org/10.5772/63927

fer steps. IPCR has been reported in detecting human interleukin 6 (IL-6) for neurological disease [95].

A further enhancement includes the immuno-RCA method that is another diagnostic platform, which utilizes DNA amplification steps to enhance the signal of immunoassay. This method employs similar concepts to IPCR but the method of DNA amplification varies. As IPCR utilizes the standard PCR amplification cycles, IRCA uses an isothermal amplification method, which does not require a thermal cycler. This makes it more attractive as there is a reduction of dependency on high-end instrumentation. IRCA was used to develop assays in detecting ovalbumin (OVA) allergens [102] and foot-and-mouth disease virus (FMDV) [103]. In IRCA, oligonucleotide primers are attached covalently to the antibody. However, DNA circularization is required to allow binding of the DNA primer to work with DNA polymerase and nucleotides for amplification to start [104]. The detection sensitivity of IRCA exceeds the conventional ELISA and microparticle formats. Thus, IRCA is a system that can allow detection of specific antigens using antibodies at high sensitivity with a wide dynamic range to detect a single molecule [104]. In short, DNA-fusion technologies with recombinant antibodies could potentially aid in the development of newer assays with improved sensitivities.

6. Conclusion

Phage display technology is commonly used for recombinant antibody production. The ability to produce antibodies via recombinant methods can help to improve the speed at which newer antibodies are produced at a fraction of the conventional cost. The freedom associated with recombinant antibodies would also allow the customization of antibodies for various downstream applications in diagnostics. This is particularly important as the development of newer technologies in sensing and reporting mechanisms, the flexibility of recombinant antibodies towards modifications would allow the antibodies to evolve with the advancement of sensing technologies. Therefore, phage display-derived recombinant antibodies provide an important platform for antibody generation for current and future diagnostic applications.

Acknowledgements

The authors would like to acknowledge support from the Malaysian Ministry of Higher Education under the HICoE program and Universiti Sains Malaysia under the Research University Individual Grant scheme (1001/CIPPM/812173).

Author details

Angela Chiew Wen Ch'ng[1,2], Yee Siew Choong[1,2] and Theam Soon Lim[1,2*]

*Address all correspondence to: theamsoon@usm.my

1 Institute for Research in Molecular Medicine, Universiti Sains Malaysia, Penang, Malaysia

2 Analytical Biochemistry Research Centre, Universiti Sains Malaysia, Penang, Malaysia

References

[1] Richman, S.A. and D.M. Kranz, *Display, engineering, and applications of antigen-specific T cell receptors.* Biomolecular Engineering, 2007. 24(4): 361–373.

[2] Alberts B. Molecular biology of the cell New York: Garland Science; 2002. Available from: http://www.ncbi.nlm.nih.gov/books/NBK21054/?depth=2.

[3] Xiong, H., et al., *E. coli expression of a soluble, active single-chain antibody variable fragment containing a nuclear localization signal.* Protein Expression and Purification, 2009. 66(2): 172–180.

[4] Cung, K., et al., *Rapid, multiplexed microfluidic phage display.* Lab on a Chip, 2012. 12(3): 562–565.

[5] Wang, J., et al., *Selection of phage-displayed peptides on live adherent cells in microfluidic channels.* Proceedings of the National Academy of Sciences, 2011. 108(17): 6909–6914.

[6] Edelman, G.M., *Antibody structure and molecular immunology.* Science, 1973. 180(88): 830–840.

[7] Becker, R.S. and K.L. Knight, *Somatic diversification of immunoglobulin heavy chain VDJ genes: evidence for somatic gene conversion in rabbits.* Cell, 1990. 63(5): 987–997.

[8] Papavasiliou, F., et al., *V (D) J recombination in mature B cells: a mechanism for altering antibody responses.* Science, 1997. 278(5336): 298–301.

[9] Searle, S., et al., *Antibody structure and function.* Antibody Engineering, 1995. 2: 3–51.

[10] Grundbacher, F., *Behring's discovery of diphtheria and tetanus antitoxins.* Immunology today, 1992. 13(5): p. 188–190.

[11] Schirrmann, T., et al., *Phage display for the generation of antibodies for proteome research, diagnostics and therapy.* Molecules, 2011. 16(1): 412–426.

[12] Emanuel, M., *Histamine and the antiallergic antihistamines: a history of their discoveries.* Clinical & Experimental Allergy, 1999. 29(S3): 1–11.

[13] Hust, M. and S. Dübel, *Phage Display Vectors for the In Vitro Generation of Human Antibody Fragments, in Immunochemical Protocols*, R. Burns, Editor. 2005, Humana Press: Totowa, NJ. p. 71–96.

[14] Hust, M., et al., *A human scFv antibody generation pipeline for proteome research.* Journal of Biotechnology, 2011. 152(4): 159–170.

[15] Karu, A.E., C.W. Bell, and T.E. Chin, *Recombinant antibody technology.* ILAR Journal, 1995. 37(3): 132–141.

[16] Carmen, S. and L. Jermutus, *Concepts in antibody phage display.* Briefings in Functional Genomics & Proteomics, 2002. 1(2): 189–203.

[17] Fukunaga, K. and M. Taki, *Practical tips for construction of custom peptide libraries and affinity selection by using commercially available phage display cloning systems.* Journal of Nucleic Acids, 2012. 2012: 9.

[18] Kretzschmar, T. and T. von Rüden, *Antibody discovery: phage display.* Current Opinion in Biotechnology, 2002. 13(6): 598–602.

[19] Levisson, M., et al., *Phage display of engineered binding proteins.* Methods in molecular biology (Clifton, NJ), 2013. 1129: p. 211–229.

[20] Li, K., et al., *A fully human scFv phage display library for rapid antibody fragment reformatting.* Protein Engineering Design and Selection, 2015: gzv024.

[21] Stricker N, Li M. Phage Display Technologies. eLS. 2001.

[22] Willats, W.G., *Phage display: practicalities and prospects.* Plant Molecular Biology, 2002. 50(6): 837–854.

[23] Beck, E. and B. Zink, *Nucleotide sequence and genome organisation of filamentous bacteriophages f1 and fd.* Gene, 1981. 16(1): 35–58.

[24] Hoogenboom, H.R., et al., *Multi-subunit proteins on the surface of filamentous phage: methodologies for displaying antibody (Fab) heavy and light chains.* Nucleic Acids Research, 1991. 19(15): 4133–4137.

[25] Qi, H., et al., *Phagemid vectors for phage display: properties, characteristics and construction.* Journal of Molecular Biology, 2012. 417(3): 129–143.

[26] Hairul Bahara, N.H., et al., *Phage display antibodies for diagnostic applications.* Biologicals, 2013. 41(4): 209–216.

[27] Lim, B.N., et al., *Principles and application of antibody libraries for infectious diseases.* Biotechnology Letters, 2014. 36(12): 2381–2392.

[28] Bakir MA, Eccles SA, Babich JW, Aftab N, Styles JM, Dean CJ, et al. *c-erbB2 Protein Overexpression in Breast Cancer as a Target for PET Using Iodine-124-Labeled Monoclonal Antibodies.* Journal of Nuclear Medicine. 1992;33(12):2154–60.

[29] Sheets, M.D., et al., *Efficient construction of a large nonimmune phage antibody library: the production of high-affinity human single-chain antibodies to protein antigens.* Proceedings of the National Academy of Sciences, 1998. 95(11): 6157–6162.

[30] Weber M, Bujak E, Putelli A, Villa A, Matasci M, Gualandi L, et al. *A Highly Functional Synthetic Phage Display Library Containing over 40 Billion Human Antibody Clones*. PLoS ONE. 2014;9(6):e100000.

[31] Sidhu, S.S. and F.A. Fellouse, *Synthetic therapeutic antibodies.* Nature Chemical Biology, 2006. 2(12): 682–688.

[32] Hoogenboom, H.R., et al., *Antibody phage display technology and its applications.* Immunotechnology, 1998. 4(1): 1–20.

[33] Benhar I. *Design of synthetic antibody libraries*. Expert Opinion on Biological Therapy. 2007;7(5):763–79.

[34] Ponsel, D., et al., *High affinity, developability and functional size: the holy grail of combinatorial antibody library generation.* Molecules, 2011. 16(5): 3675–3700.

[35] Silacci, M., et al., *Design, construction, and characterization of a large synthetic human antibody phage display library.* Proteomics, 2005. 5(9): 2340–2350.

[36] Griffiths, A.D., et al., *Isolation of high affinity human antibodies directly from large synthetic repertoires.* The EMBO Journal, 1994. 13(14): 3245.

[37] Strachan, G., et al., *Rapid selection of anti-hapten antibodies isolated from synthetic and semi-synthetic antibody phage display libraries expressed in Escherichia coli.* FEMS Microbiology Letters, 2002. 210(2): 257–261.

[38] McElhiney, J., L.A. Lawton, and A.J. Porter, *Detection and quantification of microcystins (cyanobacterialhepatotoxins) with recombinant antibody fragments isolated from a naive human phage display library.* FEMS Microbiology Letters, 2000. 193(1): 83–88.

[39] Hanes, J., et al., *Picomolar affinity antibodies from a fully synthetic naive library selected and evolved by ribosome display.* Nature Biotechnology, 2000. 18(12): 1287–1292.

[40] Rothe, C., et al., *The human combinatorial antibody library HuCAL GOLD combines diversification of all six CDRs according to the natural immune system with a novel display method for efficient selection of high-affinity antibodies.* Journal of Molecular Biology, 2008. 376(4): 1182–1200.

[41] Prassler, J., et al., *HuCAL PLATINUM, a synthetic fab library optimized for sequence diversity and superior performance in mammalian expression systems.* Journal of Molecular Biology, 2011. 413(1): 261–278.

[42] Knappik, A., et al., *Fully synthetic human combinatorial antibody libraries (HuCAL) based on modular consensus frameworks and CDRs randomized with trinucleotides.* Journal of Molecular Biology, 2000. 296(1): 57–86.

[43] Shim, H., *Synthetic approach to the generation of antibody diversity.* BMB Reports, 2015. 48(9): 489.

[44] Zebedee, S.L., et al., *Human combinatorial antibody libraries to hepatitis B surface antigen.* Proceedings of the National Academy of Sciences, 1992. 89(8): 3175–3179.

[45] Chester, K., et al., *Phage libraries for generation of clinically useful antibodies.* The Lancet, 1994. 343(8895): 455–456.

[46] Barbas, C.F. and D.R. Burton, *Selection and evolution of high-affinity human anti-viral antibodies.* Trends in Biotechnology, 1996. 14(7): 230–234.

[47] Miller, W.J., et al. *Specific immune adherence assay for human hepatitis A antibody application to diagnostic and epidemiologic investigations.* in *Proceedings of the Society for Experimental Biology and Medicine. Society for Experimental Biology and Medicine (New York, NY).* 1975.

[48] Aster, R., *Heparin induced immune thrombocytopenia–a clinical or laboratory diagnosis?* Journal of Thrombosis and Haemostasis, 2006. 4(4): 757–758.

[49] Warkentin, T. and N. Heddle, *Laboratory diagnosis of immune heparin-induced thrombocytopenia.* Current Hematology Reports, 2003. 2(2): 148–157.

[50] Mechaly, A., E. Zahavy, and M. Fisher, *Development and implementation of a single-chain Fv antibody for specific detection of Bacillus anthracis spores.* Applied and Environmental Microbiology, 2008. 74(3): 818–822.

[51] Spiliotopoulos, A., et al., *Sensitive recovery of recombinant antibody clones after their in silico identification within NGS datasets.* Journal of Immunological Methods, 2015. 420: 50–55.

[52] Kügler, J., et al., *Generation and analysis of the improved human HAL9/10 antibody phage display libraries.* BMC Biotechnology, 2015. 15(1): 10.

[53] Konthur Z, Wilde J, Lim TS. *Semi-automated Magnetic Bead-Based Antibody Selection from Phage Display Libraries.* In: Kontermann R, Dübel S, editors. Antibody Engineering. Berlin, Heidelberg: Springer Berlin Heidelberg; 2010. p. 267–287.

[54] Moreland, N.J., et al., *Phage display approaches for the isolation of monoclonal antibodies against dengue virus envelope domain III from human and mouse derived libraries.* International Journal of Molecular Sciences, 2012. 13(3): 2618–2635.

[55] Noppe, W., et al., *Chromato-panning: an efficient new mode of identifying suitable ligands from phage display libraries.* BMC Biotechnology, 2009. 9: 21–21.

[56] Kumaran J, MacKenzie CR, Arbabi-Ghahroudi M. *Semiautomated Panning of Naive Camelidae Libraries and Selection of Single-Domain Antibodies Against Peptide Antigens.* In: Saerens D, Muyldermans S, editors. Single Domain Antibodies: Methods and Protocols. Totowa, NJ: Humana Press; 2012. p. 105–24.

[57] Dias-Neto, E., et al., *Next-generation phage display: integrating and comparing available molecular tools to enable cost-effective high-throughput analysis.* PloS One, 2009. 4(12): e8338.

[58] Chin, C.F., et al., *Application of streptavidin mass spectrometric immunoassay tips for immunoaffinity based antibody phage display panning*. Journal of Microbiological Methods, 2016. 120: 6–14.

[59] Hoogenboom, H.R., et al., *Selectiondominant and nonaccessible epitopes on cell surface receptors revealed by cell-panning with a large phage antibody library*. European Journal of Biochemistry, 1999. 260(3): 774–784.

[60] Siva, A.C., et al., *Selection of anti-cancer antibodies from combinatorial libraries by whole-cell panning and stringent subtraction with human blood cells*. Journal of Immunological Methods, 2008. 330(1): 109–119.

[61] Murphy, K.M., Travers, P. and Walport, M., Janeway's *immunobiology*. New York, NY: Garland Science; 2011.

[62] Holliger, P. and P.J. Hudson, *Engineered antibody fragments and the rise of single domains*. Nature Biotechnology, 2005. 23(9): 1126–1136.

[63] Ahmad ZA, Yeap SK, Ali AM, Ho WY, Alitheen NBM, Hamid M. *scFv Antibody: Principles and Clinical Application*. Clinical and Developmental Immunology. 2012;2012:15.

[64] Hust, M. and S. Dübel, *Mating antibody phage display with proteomics*. Trends in Biotechnology, 2004. 22(1): 8–14.

[65] Holt, L.J., et al., *Domain antibodies: proteins for therapy*. Trends in Biotechnology, 2003. 21(11): 484–490.

[66] Muyldermans, S., *Single domain camel antibodies: current status*. Reviews in Molecular Biotechnology, 2001. 74(4): 277–302.

[67] Lauwereys, M., et al., *Potent enzyme inhibitors derived from dromedary heavy chain antibodies*. The EMBO Journal, 1998. 17(13): 3512–3520.

[68] Acton, Q.A., *Immunoglobulins—Advances in Research and Application: 2013 Edition*. 2013: Scholarly Editions.

[69] Chen, X., J.L. Zaro, and W.-C. Shen, *Fusion protein linkers: property, design and functionality*. Advanced Drug Delivery Reviews, 2013. 65(10): 1357–1369.

[70] Kirsch, M., et al., *Parameters affecting the display of antibodies on phage*. Journal of Immunological Methods, 2005. 301(1–2): 173–185.

[71] Lilley, G.G., et al., *Recombinant single-chain antibody peptide conjugates expressed in Escherichia coli for the rapid diagnosis of HIV*. Journal of Immunological Methods, 1994. 171(2): 211–226.

[72] Cao, M., et al., *Construction, purification, and characterization of anti-BAFF scFv–Fc fusion antibody expressed in CHO/dhfr-cells*. Applied Biochemistry and Biotechnology, 2009. 157(3): 562–574.

[73] Rau, D., K. Kramer, and B. Hock, *Single-chain Fv antibody-alkaline phosphatase fusion proteins produced by one-step cloning as rapid detection tools for ELISA.* Journal of Immunoassay and Immunochemistry, 2002. 23(2): 129–143.

[74] De Marco, A., *Strategies for successful recombinant expression of disulfide bond-dependent proteins in Escherichia coli.* Microbial Cell Factories, 2009. 8(1): 26.

[75] Beadle, C., et al., *Diagnosis of malaria by detection of Plasmodium falciparum HRP-2 antigen with a rapid dipstick antigen-capture assay.* The Lancet, 1994. 343(8897): 564–568.

[76] Moody, A., *Rapid diagnostic tests for malaria parasites.* Clinical Microbiology Reviews, 2002. 15(1): 66–78.

[77] Hu, J., et al., *Advances in paper-based point-of-care diagnostics.* Biosensors and Bioelectronics, 2014. 54: 585–597.

[78] Nahavandi, S., et al., *Microfluidic platforms for biomarker analysis.* Lab on a Chip, 2014. 14(9): 1496–1514.

[79] Lee, W.G., et al., *Nano/microfluidics for diagnosis of infectious diseases in developing countries.* Advanced Drug Delivery Reviews, 2010. 62(4): 449–457.

[80] Meagher, R.J., et al., *An integrated microfluidic platform for sensitive and rapid detection of biological toxins.* Lab on a Chip, 2008. 8(12): 2046–2053.

[81] Weigl, B., et al., *Towards non-and minimally instrumented, microfluidics-based diagnostic devices.* Lab on a Chip, 2008. 8(12): 1999–2014.

[82] Paulie, S. and H. Perlmann, *Enzyme-Linked Immunosorbent Assay, in eLS.* 2001, John Wiley & Sons, Ltd.

[83] Baptista, P., et al., *Gold nanoparticles for the development of clinical diagnosis methods.* Analytical and Bioanalytical Chemistry, 2008. 391(3): 943–950.

[84] Boisselier, E. and D. Astruc, *Gold nanoparticles in nanomedicine: preparations, imaging, diagnostics, therapies and toxicity.* Chemical Society Reviews, 2009. 38(6): 1759–1782.

[85] Thanh, N.T.K. and Z. Rosenzweig, *Development of an aggregation-based immunoassay for anti-protein A using gold nanoparticles.* Analytical Chemistry, 2002. 74(7): 1624–1628.

[86] Wilson, R., *The use of gold nanoparticles in diagnostics and detection.* Chemical Society Reviews, 2008. 37(9): 2028–2045.

[87] Posthuma-Trumpie, G.A., et al., *Amorphous carbon nanoparticles: a versatile label for rapid diagnostic (immuno) assays.* Analytical and Bioanalytical Chemistry, 2012. 402(2): 593–600.

[88] Driskell, J.D., et al., *One-step assay for detecting influenza virus using dynamic light scattering and gold nanoparticles.* Analyst, 2011. 136(15): 3083–3090.

[89] Attar, Z.J., et al., *Latex agglutination test for the detection of urinary antigens in visceral leishmaniasis.* Acta Tropica, 2001. 78(1): 11–16.

[90] Gentry, L., et al., *Latex agglutination test for detection of Candida antigen in patients with disseminated disease.* European Journal of Clinical Microbiology, 1983. 2(2): 122–128.

[91] Burnie, J. and J. Williams, *Evaluation of the Ramco latex agglutination test in the early diagnosis of systemic candidiasis.* European Journal of Clinical Microbiology, 1985. 4(2): 98–101.

[92] Kami, M., et al., *Computed tomographic scan of the chest, latex agglutination test and plasma (1AE3)-beta-D-glucan assay in early diagnosis of invasive pulmonary aspergillosis: a prospective study of 215 patients.* Haematologica, 2000. 85(7): 745–752.

[93] Westblom, T., et al., *Diagnosis of Helicobacter pylori infection in adult and pediatric patients by using Pyloriset, a rapid latex agglutination test.* Journal of Clinical Microbiology, 1992. 30(1): 96–98.

[94] Severin, W., *Latex agglutination in the diagnosis of meningococcal meningitis.* Journal of Clinical Pathology, 1972. 25(12): 1079–1082.

[95] Spengler, M., M. Adler, and C.M. Niemeyer, *Highly sensitive ligand-binding assays in pre-clinical and clinical applications: immuno-PCR and other emerging techniques.* Analyst, 2015. 140(18): 6175–6194.

[96] Breaker, R.R. and G.F. Joyce, *A DNA enzyme that cleaves RNA.* Chemistry & Biology, 1994. 1(4): 223–229.

[97] Chen, J., et al., *An ultrasensitive electrochemical biosensor for detection of DNA species related to oral cancer based on nuclease-assisted target recycling and amplification of DNAzyme.* Chemical Communications, 2011. 47(28): 8004–8006.

[98] Omar, N., et al., *Development of an antigen-DNAzymebased probe for a direct antibody-antigen assay using the intrinsic DNAzyme activity of a daunomycin aptamer.* Sensors, 2013. 14(1): 346–355.

[99] Omar, N., et al., *Development of an antigen-DNAzymebased probe for a direct antibody-antigen assay using the intrinsic DNAzyme activity of a daunomycin aptamer.* Sensors, 2014. 14: S2.

[100] Loh, Q., et al., *IQPA: Isothermal nucleic acid amplification-based immunoassay using DNAzyme as the reporter system.* Analytical Biochemistry, 2014. 463: 67–69.

[101] Malou, N. and D. Raoult, *Immuno-PCR: a promising ultrasensitive diagnostic method to detect antigens and antibodies.* Trends in Microbiology, 2011. 19(6): 295–302.

[102] Kobori, T., et al., *Rolling circle amplification for signal enhancement in ovalbumin detection.* Analytical Sciences, 2009. 25(12): 1381–1383.

[103] Van Dessel, W., et al., *Assessment of the diagnostic potential of immuno-RCA in 96-well ELISA plates for foot-and-mouth disease virus.* Journal of Virological Methods, 2008. 147(1): 151–156.

[104] Schweitzer, B., et al., *Immunoassays with rolling circle DNA amplification: a versatile platform for ultrasensitive antigen detection.* Proceedings of the National Academy of Sciences, 2000. 97(18): 10113–10119.

[105] Delaloye, B., A. Bischof-Delaloye, F. Buchegger, V. von Fliedner, J.P. Grob, J.C. Volant, et al., *Detection of colorectal carcinoma by emission-computerized tomography after injection of 123I-labeled Fab or F(ab')2 fragments from monoclonal anti-carcinoembryonic antigen antibodies.* Journal of Clinical Investigation, 1986. 77(1): 301–11.

[106] Mustafaoglu, N., N.J. Alves and B. Bilgicer, *Oriented Immobilization of Fab Fragments by Site-Specific Biotinylation at the Conserved Nucleotide Binding Site for Enhanced Antigen Detection*. Langmuir, 2015. 31(35): 9728–36.

Section 6

RDTs and Point-of-Care Testing (POCT): Quality Control, Assurance, Calibration and Safety

Chapter 8

Evaluation of Rapid Diagnostic Test Performance

Paulo Pereira

Additional information is available at the end of the chapter

http://dx.doi.org/10.5772/64179

Abstract

Rapid diagnostic tests are used for the determination of binary qualitative results not only uniquely in nonhospital-based but also in hospital-based tests. Principally, in developing countries, rapid diagnostic tests are the primary option since tests to be used in medical laboratories are discarded due to the higher cost. The test's performance is evaluated to assure that the chance of results to be false is clinically acceptable. Therefore, the diagnostic accuracy of results (diagnostic sensitivity and specificity) is assessed to guarantee the safety of postclinical decision. The statistical approach requires that representative samplings of the populations of infected and healthy individuals are tested. The area under the receiver-operating characteristic (ROC) curve is a complementary measurement using the same samplings. It represents the diagnostic accuracy in a single outcome. When samplings with known diagnostics are unavailable, samplings with known outcomes from a comparative test are used to determine the agreement of results. However, this approach is secondary, due to diagnostic accuracy to be unmeasurable. The seronegative period is another critical measurement that allows determining an individual biological bias during a period where results of an infected individual are false-negatives due to seroconversion. The claimed requirements should be defined for diagnostic accuracy and agreement outcomes. A spreadsheet is used to estimate the results considering the absolute value and the 95% confidence interval.

Keywords: clinical decision, point-of-care testing, quality assurance, quality control, rapid diagnostic test

1. Introduction

Point-of-care testing (POCT) is defined by the International Organization for Standardization (ISO) as the "testing that is performed near or at the site of the patient with the result leading to a possible change in the care of the patient" [1]. Clinical and Laboratory Standards Institute (CLSI) recognizes this definition and proposes another: "testing performed outside a central laboratory environment, generally nearer to, or at the site of the patient/client" [2]. Currently, 31% of the global *in vitro* diagnostics' (IVD) commercial tests are POCT [3]. The US POCTs represent close to 45% of the IVD market, followed by Europe and Japan. The global POCT market is estimated to increase to reach US$ 30 billion by 2020, with a compound annual growth rate close to 10% [4]. The POCT for the detection of infectious disease agents is 21.9% of the forecast POCT global market segments in 2016 [5].

Rapid diagnostic test (RDT) is one type of POCT intended to a fast detection of the antigens or antibodies present in human samples. RDT is a qualitative (or semiquantitative) test, and it is defined as the test "that detect and/or identify a particular analyte, constituent, or condition (note: this term applies to tests that detect whether a particular analyte, constituent, or condition is present or absent and sometimes assigned a positive degree (i.e., 1+, 2+)" (entry 4 in Ref. [2]). According to the International Vocabulary of Metrology (VIM), generally RDT result is analogous to nominal quantity (entry 4.26 of Ref. [6]) tests. This quantity is defined as the "rounded or approximate value of a characterizing amount of a measuring instrument or measuring system that guides its appropriate use," for example, positive/negative. Nominal quantities are sometimes confused with ordinal quantities (entry 1.26 of Ref. [6]), where a value's classification is according to a decision value on an ordinal scale, for example, a result equal or higher than the clinical decision point ("cutoff") is classified as positive, and if below —negative. RDTs are usually used as screening tests, namely, in cases where the cost per result must be lower than that if it is used in the medical laboratory test such as that happens predominantly in developing countries. They are also used when the need for an outcome is an emergent such as in an emergency room. RDT should provide accurate, precise, and reliable test results. Unreliable results have a significant probability to be untrue, affecting the clinical decision directly. According to the current good laboratory practice, RDT results should not be final results. However, in developing countries, it is frequently considered an end outcome, for what the physician should understand the risk of clinical decisions' failure due to false results. Accordingly, the laboratorian should perform a set of quality control tests to evaluate the accuracy of the RDT results. This is intended to determine and verify that the error associated to the *in vivo* results is not clinically significant (allowable error), that is, it does not affect the clinical decision significantly. When quality control tests are not performed, the residual risk (entry 2.29 of Ref. [7]) linked to the chance of incorrect clinical decisions due to abnormal results is unknown. Evidenced-based reported cases [8–11] demonstrate the impact of bad quality control practices of POCT in the clinical decisions, contributing to a discussion on the accuracy of POCT results and its association with unsafe clinical decisions [12].

Quality control (entry 3.3.7 of Ref. [13]) is a part of the quality assurance (entry 3.3.6 of Ref. [13]). It is a set of models designed to monitor the test's results. Its goal is to assure that the outcomes (true result + error) are not significantly distant from the *in vivo* results. Test evaluation should be performed determining the diagnostic accuracy of the assay focused on diagnostic sensitivity and specificity. The area under the receiver-operating characteristic curve (AUC) is a complementary measurement that permits the calculus of diagnostic uncertainty in a single outcome. Both determinations are statistical measures of the performance of a binary result (positive or negative). However, to use these applications, there must be available samplings from infected individuals D_1 and healthy individuals D_0. When the comparator is other than diagnostic, it should be determined as the agreement of results. The seronegative window period is another required measurement in an RDT evaluation. This model evaluates the seronegative period in an infected individual, during which the positive results are biologically biased, that is, they are systematically false negative.

Associated with all the presented approaches is the absence of metrological traceability of the results due to the unavailability of certified reference materials or reference methods (entry 2.41 of Ref. [6]). Therefore, RDTs are classified as untraceable tests. For a thorough discussion of metrological traceability in medical laboratories' tests, further information can be found elsewhere [14].

This chapter reviews and discusses models of diagnostic accuracy, agreement of results, and seronegative window period applied to the RDTs' evaluation. It is presented as an example a case study considering the worst scenario in a blood establishment: the use of a small number of samples where the evaluation cost must be minimum. Despite this example contributes to a less reliable estimation, its role in the consistency of the assessment remains significant. Differently from the tests' evaluation, the determination of measurement uncertainty (entry 2.26 of Ref. [3]) is not systematically applied to RDTs. However, it is considered in the estimates, considering risk-based thinking principles [15–17]. A flowchart summarizes and hierarchizes the alternatives in the selection of evaluation models. Internal quality control (entry 3.3 of Ref. [18]) and external quality assessment/proficiency testing (entry 5.1 of Ref. [19]) models are out of the chapter's scope. Ethical issues are also out of the scope. A report on legal and ethical questions of RDT is found elsewhere [20].

The theoretical principles were applied using standard spreadsheet software (Microsoft® Excel®), freely available at DOI: 10.13140/RG.2.1.1123.1766.

2. Comparison of results

2.1. Diagnostic accuracy I: 2 × 2 contingency tables

2.1.1. General concept

Diagnostic accuracy models are used to determine the RDT performance using diagnostic accuracy criteria (i.e., disease and nondisease), adopting a Bayesian probability framework. This is a concept of probability where the hypothesis of a certain condition (e.g., infected and healthy) is measured in a sampling. For this measurement, two samplings are required: one featuring infected individuals and another featuring healthy individuals. Both samples should be carefully selected to minimize the probability of sources of biological bias considerably, principally "spectrum bias." Pepe [21] defined this type of bias as the "bias between estimated test performance and true test performance when the sample used for evaluating an assay does not properly represent the entire disease spectrum over the target (intended-use) population" (entry 4.2 of Ref. [21]). The evaluator of test report recognizes there is always an estimated risk of biased results, mainly from samples of individuals in the seroconversion window period (see Section 2.4.), where the concentration of antibodies or antigens is below the RDT "cutoff." **Figure 1** illustrates the case when results of infected and healthy individuals' samples are misclassified, expressing false binary results. In this example, the results are incorrectly equal, higher or lower than the "cutoff." RDTs use a visual "cutoff" point, instead of a numerical value on an ordinal scale such as that used in diagnostic immunoassays.

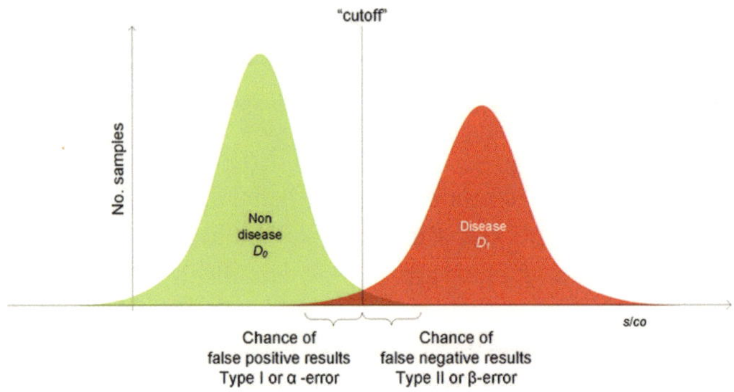

Figure 1. Classification of false results (biased results).

The performance of results is measured using diagnostic sensitivity and diagnostic specificity essentially. These terms are also recognized as clinical sensitivity, sensitivity or true positive rate and clinical specificity, specificity or true negative rate, respectively.

2.1.2. Diagnostic sensitivity

Diagnostic sensitivity *Se* [%] measures the percentage of true positive results in an infected individuals' sampling, that is, the true-positive results rate in percentage (entry 5.3 of Ref. [22]). It is determined by the mathematical model (entry 10.1.1 of Ref. [22]):

$$Se[\%] = \frac{TP}{TP + FN} \cdot 100 \quad (1)$$

where *TP* is the total of true-positive results, and *FN* is the total of false-negative results. The RDT should have a high diagnostic sensitivity to assure a nonsignificant residual risk of the erroneous clinical decision. High sensitivity suggests a high chance of true-positive results. The risk of producing false-positive or false-negative results is readily identified by the statistician to the statistical hypothesis testing as β-error or type II error or α-error or type I error, respectively. Diagnostic sensitivity is equal to $1 - FN = 1 - \beta$-error, for what it is similar to the concept of the statistical power of a binary hypothesis test (entry 2.1 of Ref. [23]), representing the capability of an assay to detect a real effect. Detailed information about statistical hypothesis tests and diagnostic accuracy tests is found elsewhere [21, 23].

The false-negative rate *FN* [%] determines the percentage of false-negative results in the infected individuals' sampling. It is referred to as "diagnostic uncertainty," since it gives a primary sense of the risk of uncertain results [24]. Consequently, "diagnostic uncertainty" of a RDT is defined as "the risk of false results." This concept is analogous to the "measurement uncertainty" intended to be applied to numerical quantity results (entry 1.20 of Ref. [6]). The determination of measurement uncertainty is demonstrated uniquely in ordinal diagnostic tests [25, 26]. In such cases, this terminology could be adapted to "measurement uncertainty of binary results." Measurement uncertainty in an RDTs' results is associated principally with the effect of between-users reading in measures of imprecision.

The false-negative rate is determined by the mathematical model (entry 10.1.4 of Ref. [22]):

$$FN[\%] = \frac{FN}{TP + FN} \cdot 100 \tag{2}$$

2.1.3. Diagnostic specificity

Diagnostic specificity *Sp* [%] measures the percentage of true-negative results in a healthy individuals' sampling, that is, the true-negative results rate in percentage (entry 5.3 of Ref. [22]). It is determined by the mathematical model (entry 10.1.1 of Ref. [22]):

$$Sp[\%] = \frac{TN}{FP + TN} \cdot 100 \tag{3}$$

where *TN* is the total of true-negative results and FP is the total of false-positive results. The false-positive rate FP [%] determines the percentage of false-positive results in the healthy individuals' sampling. In the same manner as the *FN* [%], it could be referred as "diagnostic uncertainty" [24]. It is determined by the mathematical model (entry 10.1.4 of Ref. [22]):

$$FP[\%] = \frac{FP}{FP + FN} \cdot 100 \tag{4}$$

The true and false results can be expressed in a 2 × 2 contingency table as displayed in **Table 1**.

Candidate test results	Diagnostic accuracy criteria		Total
	Positive (disease, $D = 1$)	Negative (nondisease, $D = 0$)	
Positive ($y = 1$)	True-positive results (*TP*)	False-positive results (*FP*) α-error	*TP* + *FP*
Negative ($y = 0$)	False-negative results (*FN*) β-error	True-negative results (*TN*)	*FN* + *TN*
Total	*TP* + *FN*	*FP* + *TN*	*N*

Table 1. 2 × 2 contingency table for diagnostic accuracy.

Predominantly, in rare tests, it could be difficult to have samples with an accurate diagnostic, for what comparative test results should be used when the diagnosis is unknown (see Section 2.3).

2.1.4. Inference of the results for the 95% confidence interval

The rates are applied uniquely to the sampling. They cannot be inferred to the populations. A diagnostic sensitivity equal to 100% is interpreted as a 100% probability of a result of an infected individual from the infected individuals' sampling to be a true positive. It cannot be understood as the likelihood of a person from the population of infected subjects to have a true-positive result.

Nonetheless, an inference could be used to the people of the same characteristics of sampling. Commonly, a confidence interval is used to infer to 95% of the population (95% CI), considering a risk of untrueness throughout α or β-error. To determine the 95% score confidence limits, the low limit and high limit are determined. Considering the level of trust equal to 1 – α-error, the significance level is equal to 5%. In practice, it can be statistically considered that it is 95% confident about the inclusion of true results in the interval or the error margin of 5% false results attributed to that statement.

For the diagnostic sensitivity, the low-limit interval LL_{se} and high-limit interval LL_{se} are computed from the mathematical models (entry 10.1.3 of Ref. [22]):

$$LL_{se}[\%] = \frac{Q_{1,se} - Q_{2,se}}{Q_{3,se}} \cdot 100 \tag{5}$$

$$HL_{se}[\%] = \frac{Q_{1,se} + Q_{2,se}}{Q_{3,se}} \cdot 100 \tag{6}$$

where $Q_{1,se} = 2 \cdot TP + 1.96^2$, $Q_{2,se} = 1.96 \cdot \sqrt{1.96^2 + 4 \cdot TP \cdot FN / (TP + FN)}$, and $Q_{3,se} = 2 \cdot (TP + FN + 1.96^2)$.

Low and high limits for the test's diagnostic specificity are computed, respectively, by (entry 10.1.3 of Ref. [22])

$$LL_{sp}[\%] = \frac{Q_{1,sp} - Q_{2,sp}}{Q_{3,sp}} \cdot 100 \tag{7}$$

$$HL_{sp}[\%] = \frac{Q_{1,sp} - Q_{2,sp}}{Q_{3,sp}} \cdot 100 \tag{8}$$

where $Q_{1,sp} = 2 \cdot TN + 1.96^2$; $Q_{2,se} = 1.96 \cdot \sqrt{1.96^2 + 4 \cdot FP \cdot TN / (FP + TN)}$, and $Q_{3,sp} = 2 \cdot (FP + TN + 1.96^2)$.

2.1.5. Overall accuracy

Efficiency is an overall estimation of the accuracy in the samplings expressing the percentage of true results in the total of results (entry 4 of Ref. [27]). It is determined by the mathematical model (entry 9.1 of Ref. [27]):

$$Eff[\%] = \frac{TP + TN}{N} \cdot 100 \tag{9}$$

2.1.6. Predictive values

The prediction value of negative results, positive results, or both in a sampling or population has interested the clinical field. Physicians may wish to know the probability of true result to be associated with the presence or absence of a disease, and these can be provided easily.

Predictive value of a positive result or positive predictive value *PPV* [%] measures the percentage of infected individuals in the positive results sampling (entry 5.3 of Ref. [22]). It is determined by the mathematical model (entry 10.3.1 of Ref. [22]):

$$PPV[\%] = \frac{TP}{TP + FP} \cdot 100 \tag{10}$$

Predictive value of a negative result or negative predictive value *NPV* [%] measures the percentage of healthy individuals in the negative results sampling (entry 5.3 of Ref. [22]). It is determined by the mathematical model (entry 10.3.1 of Ref. [22]):

$$NPV[\%] = \frac{TN}{TN + FN} \cdot 100 \tag{11}$$

2.1.7. Prevalence of infected individuals' sampling

Prevalence is not an indicator of performance, but an indicator of the frequency of infected individuals' samples in the total number of subjects. Prevalence of infected individuals *Pr* [%] measures the percentage of infected persons in the total of tested subjects (entry 5.3 of Ref. [22]). It is determined by the mathematical model (entry 10.3.1 of Ref. [22]):

$$Pr[\%] = \frac{TP + FN}{N} \cdot 100 \tag{12}$$

2.1.8. Reproducibility conditions of the study

The sample's measurement should occur in reproducibility conditions, to assure the study evaluates the major error components of the test. For example, if the RDT is to be used by more than one user, it should be tested by all, or if unfeasible, by a representative sampling. Usually, it is recommended the evaluation take place in a period during 10–20 days (entry 9.3 of Ref. [22]). This period is understood as the time when all significant causes of error are expected to happen. However, batch-to-batch variation is commonly omitted, which requires that each batch should be evaluated independently. Sometimes, the evaluations of different batches are done by the inference of one batch's evaluation, which is statistically incorrect since a single batch is not representative of a reagent's manufacturer production.

2.1.9. Interference of results

The samples should be verified taking into account the causes of pre-analytical interference to minimize the risk of false results, biasing diagnostic sensitivity and specificity results. The contribution to false results of anticoagulant, bilirubin, erythrocytes, hemoglobin, dialysis [28], disease effects [29], drugs' effects [30], herbs, and natural products is recognized [31]. The laboratorian could identify the documented interference in published literature or the manufacturer's paper inserted in the reagent kit.

2.1.10. Re-evaluation

The RDT re-evaluation should occur principally when significant epidemiological changes happen; however, other changes require a re-evaluation such as the alteration of the users or even a change in the reagent batch.

2.2. Diagnostic accuracy II: area under the receiver operating characteristic curve

2.2.1. Receiver operating characteristic curve

ROC curve could be defined as "a graphical description of test performance representing the relationship between the diagnostic sensitivity and the false-positive rate" (entry 4.2 of Ref. [32]). **Figure 2** shows three ROC curves. ROC A assures 100% true results using infinite number of determinations from samplings of infected and healthy individuals, which is an unrealistic case; ROC B assumes a realistic situation where a negligible probability of false result happens; and ROC C assures 100% true false results, which is an unrealistic example. A curve following closer to the left-hand border and then the top border represents accurate test's results. ROC is purely a graphical plot exhibiting the performance of an assay as the "cutoff" differs. Accordingly, its application to the RDT user is hard to apply, since there is no numerical "cutoff" but uniquely a visual "cutoff," which cannot be expressed as a numerical quantity by the user. A semiquantitative classification such as a positive degree is not applied usually to these tests.

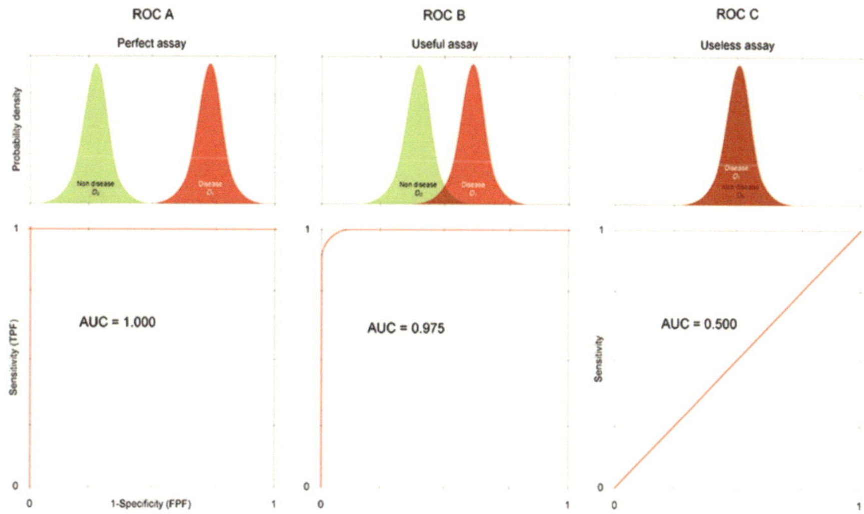

Figure 2. Three hypothetical ROC curves.

2.2.2. *Area under the receiver operating characteristic curve*

The area under the receiver operating characteristic curve (AUC) determines the ability of a test to classify accurately or discriminate samples. It ranges from 0.5 to 1, signifying respectively, binary results randomly assigned to a sample and a perfect test discrimination. It could be measured using parametric or nonparametric models [24], such as the D'Agostino-Pearson normality test AUC_p [33] and the Mann-Whitney U statistical test AUC_{np} [34], correspondingly. Both models could be computed using the data previously requested in Section 2.1.:

$$AUC_p = FPF(c) \cdot TPF(c) \tag{13}$$

where $FPF(c)$ is the false-positive rate for a defined "cutoff" value c and $TPF(c)$ is the true-positive rate for the same "cutoff" [35].

$$AUC_{np} = U / n_1 \cdot n_0 \tag{14}$$

where $U = (n_1 \cdot n_0 + n_0 \cdot (n_0 + 1))/(2 - R)$, where R is the rank sum of squares; n_1 is the number of negative specimens; and n_0 is the number of positive samples [34].

The difference between one and the AUC could also be referred as "diagnostic uncertainty" of estimation.

Test discrimination could be classified according to the AUC, using the following ratings [36]:

- if $AUC \in [0.50, 0.70]$ the distinction is poor;

- if $AUC \in [0.70, 0.80]$ the distinction is acceptable;
- if $AUC \in [0.80, 0.90]$ the distinction is excellent;
- and if $AUC \in [0.90, 1.00]$ the distinction is outstanding.

The accuracy of AUC is restricted by the number of true and false results. It gives an overall evaluation of RDT performance, complementing diagnostic sensitivity and specificity estimates [24]. As in Section 2.1.4, a confidence interval should be related to the AUC to evaluate if changes in AUC between classifiers are statistically significant in the inferred range. The report evaluator could erroneously infer about the capacity of an RDT to discriminate the results if the absolute values are considered uniquely. The 95% CI could be computed according to the model

$$AUC \pm 1.96 \cdot \mathrm{SE[AUC]} \tag{15}$$

Where SE[AUC] is the standard error determination of the AUC which is computed by Var[TP]/n_1+Var[FP]/n_2 where Var[TP] is the variance of true positive results,$n_1$is the number of true positive results, Var[FP] is the variance of false positive results, and n_2 is the number of false positive results [37]. Despite apparently it has the advantage of the results to be centered on the absolute value, it was not recommended by Newcombe [38], claiming the feature of symmetry leads to an uncorrected calculus due to "overshoot" and "degeneracy." Newcombe suggested the Clopper-Pearson model for calculating exact binomial confidence intervals, used to the 95% CI determination, eliminating the incidence of both defects. The model contemplates the interval $[AUC_{LL}, AUC_{HL}]$ with $AUC_{LL} \leq p \leq AUC_{HL}$, such that for all θ in the interval:

$$if\ AUC_{LL} \leq \theta \leq p, kp_r + \Sigma_{j:r<j\leq n} p_{j\geq \alpha/2}; \text{and} \tag{16}$$

$$if\ p \leq \theta \leq AUC_{HL}, kp_r + \Sigma_{j:0\leq j<n} p_j + kp_{r\geq \alpha/2} \tag{17}$$

where $j = 0, 1,\ldots, n$, R representing the random variable of which r is the realization, and $k = 1$ [39].

The significance level is equal to 5%, and it is another analogy to "diagnostic uncertainty" (see Section 2.1.4).

Since the AUC depends primarily on the number of true and false results, it is determined in RDT, considering the used "cutoff" exclusively.

2.2.3. *Reproducibility, interferences, and re-evaluation*

The reproducibility conditions, the interferences, and the re-evaluation are considered as seen in Sections 2.1.8, 2.1.9, and 2.1.10, respectively.

2.3. Agreement of binary results when comparator is other than diagnostic accuracy criteria

2.3.1. General concept

The principles used in Section 2.1 to compute the rates are not applicable to the determination of agreement between results of a candidate RDT and a comparative test. Despite the mathematical models being similar, the diagnostic accuracy is unmeasurable since the individuals' diagnostic is unidentified. It classifies merely the concordance of results. In this model, the diagnostic is replaced by the outcome of a comparative test different from a "gold standard" test [22]. The comparative test should have an acceptable diagnostic accuracy to minimize bias. When there is only available a comparative test without acknowledged diagnostic accuracy, the risk of bias effect in concordance is major, which could signify the agreements' results are unrealistic when compared to diagnostic accuracy. For example, this case happens if the comparative test's diagnostic accuracy is lower than that in the candidate RDT. In this condition, a nonconcordance could be erroneously interpreted. The evaluation is also erroneous when the agreement concept is misinterpreted as diagnostic accuracy.

Table 2 summarizes the agreement of binary results and the α and β errors.

Candidate test results	Comparative test		Total
	Positive ($x = 1$)	Negative ($x = 0$)	
Positive ($y = 1$)	Positive agreement (a)	Negative disagreement (b), α-error	$a + b$
Negative ($y = 0$)	Positive disagreement (c), β-error	Negative agreement (d)	$c + d$
Total	$a + c$	$b + d$	n

Table 2. 2 × 2 contingency table for test results agreement.

2.3.2. Agreement of overall results

The percentage of positive and negative results agreement is designated "overall percent agreement" *OPA* [%], and it is computed by (entry 10.2.1 of Ref. 22])

$$OPA[\%] = \frac{a + d}{n} \cdot 100 \tag{18}$$

where a is the total of candidate test's positive results among the positive results of the comparative test, d is the total of candidate test's negative outcomes among the negative results in the comparative test, and n is the total number of samples.

2.3.3. Agreement of positive results

The percentage of positive results agreement is designated "positive percent agreement" *PPA* [%], and it is computed by (entry 10.2.1 of Ref. [22])

$$PPA[\%] = \frac{a}{a+c} \cdot 100 \tag{19}$$

2.3.4. Agreement of negative results

The percentage of negative results agreement is designated "negative percent agreement" *NPA* [%], and it is computed by (entry 10.2.1 of Ref. [22])

$$NPA[\%] = \frac{d}{b+d} \cdot 100 \tag{20}$$

2.3.5. Inference of the results for the 95% confidence interval

Such as in the diagnostic accuracy (see Section 2.1.4) to infer an estimation to the population, a 95% confidence interval is used. Accordingly, the low and high limits for the test's overall percent agreement are computed respectively by (entry 10.2.2 of Ref. [22])

$$LL_{OPA}[\%] = \frac{Q_{1,OPA} - Q_{2,OPA}}{Q_{3,OPA}} \cdot 100 \tag{21}$$

$$HL_{OPA}[\%] = \frac{Q_{1,OPA} + Q_{2,OPA}}{Q_{3,OPA}} \cdot 100 \tag{22}$$

where $Q_{1,OPA} = 2 \cdot (a+d) + 1.96^2$, $Q_{2,OPA} = 1.96 \cdot \sqrt{1.96^2 + 4 \cdot (a+d) \cdot (b+c) / n}$ and $Q_{3,OPA} = 2 \cdot (n + 1.96^2)$.

Low and high limits for the test's positive percent agreement are computed respectively by (entry 10.2.2 of Ref. [22])

$$LL_{PPA}[\%] = \frac{Q_{1,PPA} - Q_{2,PPA}}{Q_{3,PPA}} \cdot 100 \tag{23}$$

$$HL_{PPA}[\%] = \frac{Q_{1,PPA} + Q_{2,PPA}}{Q_{3,PPA}} \cdot 100 \tag{24}$$

where $Q_{1,PPA} = 2 \cdot a + 1.96^2$, $Q_{2,PPA} = 1.96 \cdot \sqrt{1.96^2 + 4 \cdot a \cdot c / (a+c)}$, and $Q_{3,PPA} = 2 \cdot (a + c + 1.96^2)$.

Low and high limits for the test's negative percent agreement are computed, respectively, by (entry 10.2.2 of Ref. [22])

http://dx.doi.org/10.5772/64179

$$LL_{NPA}[\%] = \frac{Q_{1,NPA} - Q_{2,NPA}}{Q_{3,NPA}} \cdot 100 \tag{25}$$

$$HL_{NPA}[\%] = \frac{Q_{1,NPA} - Q_{2,NPA}}{Q_{3,NPA}} \cdot 100 \tag{26}$$

where $Q_{1,NPA} = 2 \cdot d + 1.96^2$, $Q_{2,NPA} = 1.96 \cdot \sqrt{1.96^2 + 4 \cdot b \cdot d / (b + d)}$, and $Q_{3,NPA} = 2 \cdot (b + d + 1.96^2)$ (note: a, b, c, and d are analogous to the number of "true positives," "false positives," "false negatives," and "true negatives" results of diagnostic accuracy).

The significance level is equal to 5%, and it is another time analogous to "diagnostic uncertainty." The claimed confidence interval should take into consideration the same limitations associated with the selection of intervals also discussed in Section 2.1.4.

2.3.6. *Reproducibility and interferences*

The reproducibility conditions and the interferences are treated as seen in Sections 2.1.8 and 2.1.9, respectively.

2.3.7. *Re-evaluation*

The RDT re-evaluation should take place mainly when significant epidemiological changes happen, and the comparative test is re-evaluated. As seen in Section 2.1.10, the variations in the batch of the reagent also involve re-evaluation study.

2.4. Seroconversion window period

2.4.1. *General concept*

The seroconversion window period is also recognized as the "seronegative period" or the "seroconversion sensitivity" [40]. Seroconversion period is defined as "the window period for a test designed to detect a specific disease (particularly an infectious disease) is the time between first infection and when the test can reliably detect that infection" [41]. The window period is equal to the number of days starting on the day of infection (day zero) to the day of the first positive result, that is, the time taken for seroconversion. Pereira et al. [42] proposed an alternative definition considering a trinary classification (i.e., positive/indeterminate/negative), which is uniquely applicable to tests with an ordinal scale of results.

2.4.2. *Seronegative period*

The evaluation of a seroconversion panel allows a primary determination of the most critical source of bias (biological bias), that is, the seronegative period. It is the major component of the risk of the incorrect clinical decision [39]. The window period is also a diagnostic accuracy test despite not commonly classified as such to distinguish from Bayesian models (see Section 2.1).

The window period performance differs according to the type and the generation of the test. It depends also on the seroconversion panel used, which represents a unique infected individual and cannot be inferred to all the people with risk behaviors. Consequently, this period cannot be related to all the seronegative persons. It should not be misunderstood as the window period of a test, which is unknown. A benchmarking study should consider the shortest period in a rank of tests for comparison, usually coming with inserted literature in seroconversion panel.

For an in-depth discussion of seroconversion window period, further information can be found elsewhere [43].

2.4.3. Re-evaluation

The re-evaluation should only occur when a new panel with a shorter period is available. The laboratorian should consult the updated list of obtainable panels in the websites of manufacturers or the published literature.

3. Results and discussion

3.1. A case study

A practical example of the use of RDT results is in the evaluation of human blood components in a blood establishment (blood bank). In this case, the selection of the infected individuals should take into consideration the epidemiological prevalence not only of the tested agent but also types, subtypes, and other variants of significant epidemiological prevalence in the geographic area of the candidates to blood donors. If the sampling does not feature all the epidemiological significant variants, the diagnostic sensitivity is biased, and the results of the new variants are inaccurate. Otherwise, the selection of healthy individuals' sampling should include uniquely subjects recognized as noninfected. The regular blood donors' population is the best source for sampling of healthy subjects, since they are clinical and laboratory screened during a long term.

3.2. The rapid diagnostic test

To exemplify the models is used a single commercial RDT to detect antihuman immunodeficiency virus types 1 (HIV-1) and 2 (HIV-2) antibodies in human serum, plasma, venous blood, and capillary blood. Since it is to be used uniquely with serum, the evaluation occurs using serum specimens. The recombinant antigens (HIV-1 gp120, gp41, and HIV-2 gp36) conjugated to colloidal gold are adsorbed on a base of a strip of nitrocellulose membrane. There are two test zones: (1) test zone, where HIV-1 and HIV-2 antigens are immobilized, and (2) control zone, where anti-HIV antibodies are immobilized. For internal quality control of the test is used a control zone. Interpret results as follows: there is no red strip in the test zone when the antibodies anti-HIV-1 or anti-HIV-2 are immeasurable, and there is a red strip in the control zone due to the migration of the antigen-conjugate gold (negative result). If the antibodies anti-HIV-1 or anti-HIV-2 are measurable, both zones have a red strip (positive result). Whenever the control zone does not have a red strip, the results do not have a binary classification (unclassified results). Repetitive positive must be tested using a confirmatory test, such as Western Blot, for antibodies.

3.3. Diagnostic accuracy I: 2 × 2 contingency tables

The evaluation contemplates a worst case considering:

- The laboratorians are trained successfully;
- The assessment is performed in a short period in reproducibility condition;
- The number of samples of infected individuals and healthy individuals is minor to assure a low cost of the assessment and to be feasible for a short period;
- The intended use of the RDT results is the screening of individuals with risk behavior to HIV infection.

Considering the major problem to a clinical decision to be false-negative outcomes, a larger number of infected individuals' samples is selected ($n = 10$), when compared to the number of healthy individuals ($n = 5$). The performance focuses on diagnostic sensitivity instead of diagnostic specificity. The samples are from diagnosed patients infected with HIV-1 ($n = 9$) and HIV-2 ($n = 1$), with repeated positive results to a fourth generation chemiluminescence immunoassay, Western Blot, and nucleic acid test (reverse transcription-polymerase chain reaction). Healthy subjects are regular blood donors tested in last three blood donations, with successive negative results to a fourth generation chemiluminescence immunoassay. The HIV group of the tested samples is not classified.

The claimed performance is determined according to the manufacturer's literature and the number of samples. When a 95% CI minimum requirement is claimed, the number of samples must be considered, since it is a restriction of the claim. Requested performance for absolute results is equal to 100% to diagnostic sensitivity and 90% to diagnostic specificity. The best diagnostic sensitivity's low limit is equal to 72.2%, and diagnostic specificity's low limit is equal to 56.6%, which is useless for the evaluation. In this case, the 95% CI is considered only to diagnostic sensitivity, since the minor number of healthy individuals' samples does not assure a reliable estimate. The lower limit of 95% CI of the claimed diagnostic sensitivity is 65%.

	Samples [*n*]		[%]							
	D_1	D_0	*Se*	*FNR*	*Sp*	*FPR*	*Eff*	*PPV*	*NPV*	*Pr*
Absolute	10	5	100	0	100	0	100	100	100	66.7
95% CI	–	–	72.2–100	–	56.6–100	–	–	–	–	–

Table 3. Number of samples and diagnostic accuracy of binary results.

Table 3 shows the performance rates to the candidate RDT, demonstrating that the requirements have been achieved with an overall accuracy of the test equal to 100%. **Figure 3** displays the true and false results in a three-dimensional data chart. The diameters of the disks are proportional to the number of outcomes. Despite the prevalence rates are unusable to the test evaluation, they could be useful to support the clinical decisions by the physician.

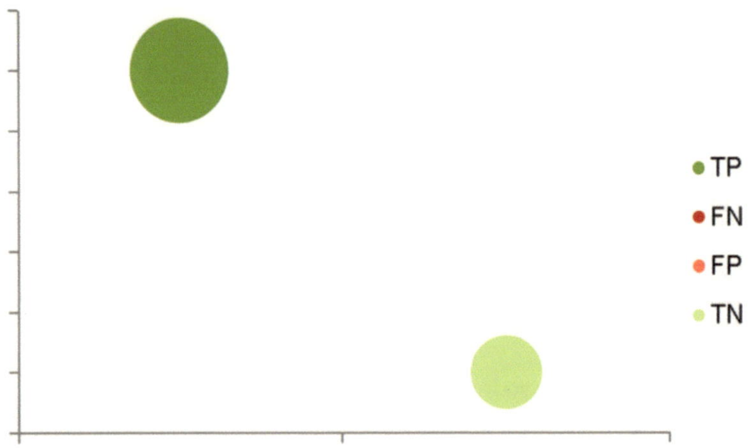

Figure 3. Bubble chart for the diagnostic uncertainty outcomes: true-positive (TP), false-negative (FN), false-positive (FP), and true-negative (TN) results.

It can be described that all samples of infected individuals and healthy individuals reported true results, and can be statistically considered that it is 95% confident about the inclusion of true-positive results in the interval or the error margin of 5% false-negative results attributed to that statement. The 95% CI can be interpreted as the diagnostic accuracy range.

The predictive value of positive and negative results is equal. This is interpreted as the samplings' results are accurately associated to the diagnostic.

3.4. Diagnostic accuracy II: receiver operating characteristic curve

The same data is used to determine the AUC as in the previous model. The AUC is computed using the Clopper-Pearson nonparametric method described above, since the hypothesis of the normal distribution of test results could not be tested. Claimed absolute value is 1.00 and the claimed 95% CI is [0.75, 1.00].

http://dx.doi.org/10.5772/64179

The AUC absolute value is 1.00, ranking the RDT as an "outstanding discrimination" test, with a 95% CI equal to [0.78, 1.00], whereby the RDT's AUC is accepted. It can be considered statistically that it is 95% confident about the inclusion of true results in the interval or the error margin of 5% false results attributed to that statement. Such as in Section 2.1.4., the 95% CI can be understood as the diagnostic accuracy interval. As it was already discussed, the AUC interpretation considers that the low limit is influenced by the number of samples tested. A minor number of samples decreases the statistical power of the evaluation, making its use unreliable.

These calculi are also useful for the definition of "cutoff" point in an RDT in the research and development phase. The "cutoff" is selected considering mainly its impact on the diagnostic sensitivity and specificity according to results' intended use, that could be interpreted as the adequation of the diagnostic sensitivity and specificity according to its role in the clinical decision. The measurements needed to plot the ROC curve are essential for manufacturers of *in vitro* diagnostics medical devices to determine the "cutoff" value for a test under development. This is also appropriate such as for medical laboratory "in house" and "nonwaived" modified tests (entry 42 CFR Subparts H, J, K and M of Ref. [44]), where the "cutoff" must be identified. The AUC single value is applicable only to the samplings of infected and healthy individuals, and it cannot be related to the population groups. For example, the "cutoff" point as a result of $AUC = 1.00$ divides perfectly the two groups, but it is unknown if it divides the two groups in the population. Then, the AUC 95% CI is determined since it is an inference to the population characterized in the same manner as the tested sampling. When the population has unlike characteristics than the sampling, the 95% CI is biased. The AUC utility, when applied to RDT evaluation in practice, is limited to represent the diagnostic test's accuracy in a single value, complementing diagnostic sensitivity and specificity results.

3.5. Agreement of binary results when comparator is other than diagnostic accuracy criteria

The same samplings as that in the previous models are used. They are also tested in a comparator test; in this example, a second RDT. Claimed requirements determine rates to be equal to 100% to the overall, positive, and negative agreements. The 95% score low confidence limit is claimed to be equal or higher than 70% to the overall and positive agreements. Such as in the 95% CI of diagnostic specificity, the confidence interval is not considered to the negative agreement. **Table 4** displays the estimates of results' agreement, showing that only the PPA result is achieved to the absolute and confidence interval. It can be statistically considered that it is 95% confident about the inclusion of agreements in the interval or the error margin of 5% disagreements attributed to that statement. In this case, the overall and negative agreements results were influenced by one false-negative result of the comparator test. This is an example of a major inaccuracy (bias) due to the use of a comparator with a weak performance (poor diagnostic specificity) when compared to candidate test. This evaluation approach should be only used exceptionally when the diagnosis is unspecified. The evaluator should use further studies to verify if the inaccurate results are due to the candidate's or comparator's test performance, to reduce the risk of erroneous conclusions.

	Samples [*n*]				
	Positive	Negative	*OPA* [%]	*PPA* [%]	*NPA* [%]
Absolute	10	5	93.3	100	83.3
95% CI	–	–	70.2–98.8	70.1–100	43.6–97.0

Table 4. Number of samples and agreement of binary results.

3.6. Seroconversion window period

The Window period estimate is performed with a seropositive commercial panel. The panel contains six undiluted and unpreserved plasma samples of an infected 19-year-old male. The manufacturer does not feature any RDT result in the inserted paper. **Figure 4** shows that 12 days after the first bleed, the RDT can detect the presence of HIV-1 antibodies reliably. Panel manufacturer inserted paper demonstrates that HIV RNA (copies/mL) is detected on the first day of bleed in one test in a series of two. Positive results are determined on the fifth day in three fourth generation immunoassays (detecting HIV-1 and HIV-2 antibodies, and HIV-1 p24 antigen) in a series of six tests. In a series of five antibody immunoassays, all have positive results after the 12th day. Thus, the RDT window period is equivalent to the tests to antibodies in this panel. As predictable, the window period was shorter in immunoassays also detecting HIV-1 p24 antigen and even shorter in nucleic acid tests. Such happens with any other test; a confirmatory scheme should be used to establish positive final results in RDT.

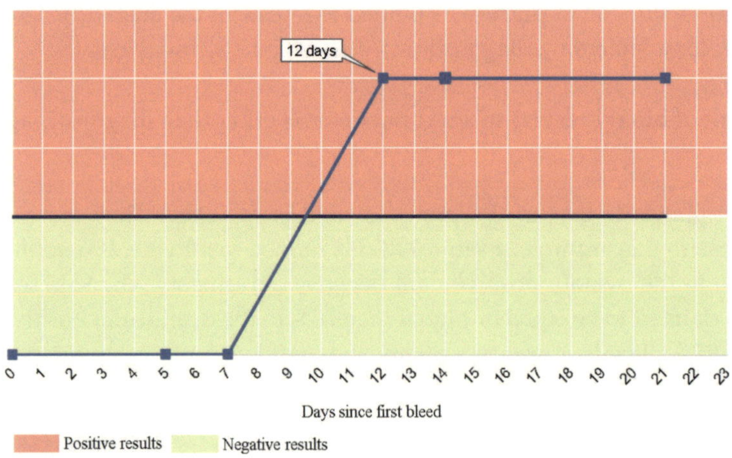

Figure 4. Results over time from six samples of a seroconversion commercial panel from a plasma donor who seroconverted over the course of their donation history.

3.7. Recommended flowchart

The selection and practical application of the evaluation models are summarized in a flowchart displayed in **Figure 5**.

http://dx.doi.org/10.5772/64179

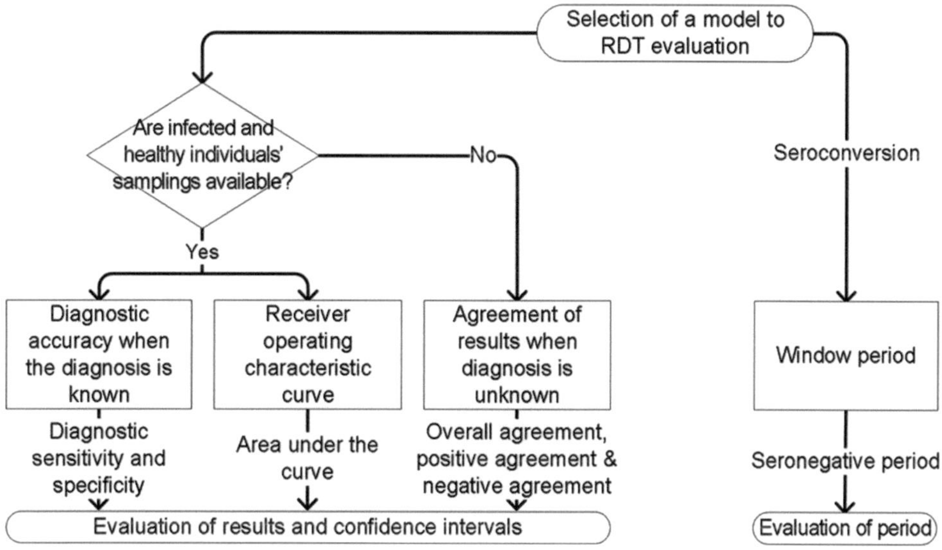

Figure 5. Flowchart to the selection of models to evaluate a RDT.

4. Conclusion

Summarizing, the diagnostic accuracy of RDT characterizes the level of confidence of binary results to be accurate (true) and the significance standards of a confidence interval. The determination of agreement of results is usually not a reliable estimate, for what its estimation should occur only when there is no possible to test samples with known diagnostic. The AUC is merely complementary to the diagnostic sensitivity and specificity evaluations. The seronegative window period is determined to evaluate an approximate period where false-negative results occur due to the antibodies' concentration being unmeasurable. This is expected in populations with a high epidemiological prevalence of tested agent. Such as in any other test, results have a chance to be untrue, whereby the physician should consider the predictive value of results during the clinical decisions based on the reported results.

Author details

Paulo Pereira

Address all correspondence to: paulo.pereira@ipst.min-saude.pt

Quality Management Department, Portuguese Institute of Blood and Transplantation, Lisbon, Portugal

References

[1] International Organization for Standardization. ISO 22870 Point-of-care testing (POCT)—Requirements for quality and competence. Geneva: ISO; 2006.

[2] Clinical and Laboratory Standards Institute. POCT04-A2 Point-of-care in vitro diagnostic (IVD) testing. 2nd ed. Wayne (PA): CLSI; 2006.

[3] Witonsky J. BioMarket Trends, IVD market moving rapidly on an upward trajectory. Genet Eng Biotechn 2015, 32(21):14–14. DOI: 10.1089/gen.32.21.05

[4] Reuters. Press release: Research and markets: Global point-of-care diagnostics market outlook 2014-2018—United States accounts for almost 50% of total market. Retrieved from: http://www.reuters.com/article/research-and-markets-idUSnBw206639a+100+BSW20140520. Accessed: March 26, 2016.

[5] Frost & Sullivan. NE3E-01 Analysis of the Global In Vitro Diagnostics Market. Retrieved from: http://www.frost.com/sublib/display-report.do?id=NE3E-01-00-00-00. Accessed: March 26, 2016.

[6] Bureau International des Poids et Mesures. JCGM 200:2012 International vocabulary of metrology—Basic and general concepts and associated terms, 2008 version with minor corrections. 3rd ed. Sèvres: BIPM; 2012. Retrieved from: http://www.bipm.org/utils/common/documents/jcgm/JCGM_200_2012.pdf. Accessed: March 26, 2016.

[7] International Organization for Standardization. ISO 31000 Risk management—Principles and guidelines. Geneva: ISO; 2009.

[8] Renaud B, Maison P, Ngako A, Cunin P, Santin A, et al. Impact of point-of-care testing in the emergency department evaluation and treatment of patients with suspected acute coronary syndromes. Acad Emerg Med 2008, 15(3):216–224. DOI: 10.1111/j.1553-2712.2008.00069.x

[9] Takakuwa K, Ou FS, Peterson E, Pollack, C, Jr, Peacock F, et al. The usage patterns of cardiac bedside markers employing point-of-care testing for troponin in non-ST-segment elevation acute coronary syndrome: Results from CRUSADE. Clin Cardiol 2009, 32(9):498–505. DOI: 10.1002/clc.20626

[10] Arias C, Panesso D, McGrath D, Qin X, Mojica M, et al. Rivaroxaban versus warfarin in nonvalvular atrial fibrillation. N Engl J Med 2011, 365(10):892–900. DOI: 10.1056/NEJMoa1009638

[11] Cohen D. Rivaroxaban: Can we trust the evidence? BMJ 2016, 352(i575):1–4. DOI: 10.1136/bmj.i575

[12] Van Hoof V. Quality in point-of-care testing. (How) can the quality of POCT results be guaranteed? In: Antwerp TQM conference; March 14 and 15, 2016; Belgium.

[13] International Organization for Standardization. ISO 9000 Quality management systems —Fundamentals and vocabulary. 4th ed. Geneva: ISO; 2015.

[14] Vesper H, Thienpont L. Traceability in laboratory medicine. Clin Chem 2009, 55(6): 1067–1075. DOI: 10.1373/clinchem.2008.107052

[15] Pereira P, Westgard J, Encarnação P, Seghatchian J, Sousa G. Quality management in the European screening laboratories in blood establishments: A view on current approaches and trends. Transfus Apher Sci 2015, 52(2):245–251. DOI: 10.1016/j.transci.2015.02.014

[16] Pereira P, Westgard J, Encarnação P, Seghatchian J, de Sousa G. The role of uncertainty in results of screening immunoassays in blood establishments. Transfus Apher Sci 2015, 52(2):252–255. DOI: 10.1016/j.transci.2015.02.015

[17] International Organization for Standardization. ISO 9001 Quality management systems —Requirements. 5th ed. Geneva: ISO; 2015.

[18] Clinical and Laboratory Standards Institute. EP29-A Expression of measurement uncertainty in laboratory medicine. Wayne (PA): CLSI; 2012.

[19] Clinical and Laboratory Standards Institute. H43-A2 Clinical flow cytometric analysis of neoplastic hematolymphoid cells. 2nd ed. Wayne (PA): CLSI; 2007.

[20] Elliott R, Jürgens R. Rapid HIV screening at the point of care: Legal and ethical questions. Canadian HIV/AIDS Legal Network; 2000. Retrieved from: http://www.aidslaw.ca/site/download/9359/. Accessed: March 26, 2016.

[21] Pepe M. The Statistical evaluation of medical tests for classification and prediction. Oxford: Oxford University Press; 2004.

[22] Clinical and Laboratory Standards Institute. EP12-A2 User protocol for evaluation of qualitative test performance. 2nd ed. Wayne (PA): CLSI; 2008.

[23] Zhou X, Obuchowski N, McCLish D. Statistical methods in diagnostic medicine. 2nd ed. Hoboken (NJ): John Wiley & Sons; 2002.

[24] Pereira P, Westgard J, Encarnação P, Seghatchian J. Evaluation of the measurement uncertainty in screening immunoassays in blood establishments: Computation of diagnostic accuracy models. Transfus Apher Sci 2015, 52(1):35–41. DOI: 10.1016/j.transci.2014.12.017

[25] Pereira P, Magnusson B, Theodorsson E, Westgard J, Encarnação P. Measurement uncertainty as a tool for evaluating the "grey-zone" to reduce the false negatives in immunochemical screening of blood donors for infectious diseases. Accred Qual Assur 2016, 21(1):25–32. DOI: 10.1007/s00769-015-1180-x

[26] Pereira P. Uncertainty of measurement in medical laboratories. In: Cocco L, editor. Measurement systems. Rijeka: InTech; 2016.

[27] Clinical and Laboratory Standards Institute. EP12-A User protocol for evaluation of qualitative test performance. Wayne (PA): CLSI; 2002.

[28] Young D. Effects of drugs on clinical laboratory tests. Volumes 1 & 2. 5th ed. Washington (DC): AACC Press; 2000.

[29] Young D. Effects of Disease on Clinical Laboratory Tests. Volumes 1 & 2. 4th ed. Washington (DC): AACC Press; 2001.

[30] Young D. Effects of Preanalytical Variables on Clinical Laboratory Tests. 3rd ed. Washington (DC): AACC Press; 2007.

[31] Narayanan S, Young D. Effects of herbs and natural products on clinical laboratory tests. Washington (DC): AACC Press; 2007.

[32] Clinical and Laboratory Standards Institute. EP24-A2 Assessment of the clinical accuracy of laboratory tests using receiver operating characteristic curves. 2nd ed. Wayne (PA): CLSI; 2011.

[33] D'Agostino RB, Belanger A, D'Agostino RB Jr. A suggestion for using powerful and informative tests of normality. Am Stat 1990, 44(4):316–321. DOI: 10.2307/2684359

[34] Mann H, Whitney D. On a test of whether one of two random variables is stochastically larger than the other. Ann Math Stat 1947, 18(1):50–60. DOI:10.1214/aoms/1177730491

[35] Metz C. Basic principles of ROC analysis. Semin Nucl Med 1978, 8(4):283–298. DOI: 10.1016/S0001-2998(78)80014-2

[36] Hosmer D, Jr, Lemeshow S, Sturdivant R. Assessing the fit of the model. In: Hosmer D Jr, Lemeshow S, Sturdivant R, editors. Solutions manual to accompany applied logistic regression. 2nd ed. Hoboken (NJ): John Wiley & Sons, 2013; p. 153–226.

[37] DeLong E, DeLong D, Clarke-Pearson D. Comparing the area under two or more correlated receiver operating characteristic curves: a nonparametric approach. Biometrics 1988, 44(3):837–45. DOI: 10.2307/2531595

[38] Newcombe R. Two sided confidence intervals for the single proportion: A comparative evaluation of seven methods. Stat Med 1998, 17(8):857–872. DOI: 10.1002/(SICI)1097-0258(19980430)17:8<857::AID-SIM777>3.0.CO;2-E

[39] Clopper CJ, Pearson ES. The use of confidence or fiducial limits illustrated in the case of the binomial. Biometrika 1934, 26(4):404–413. DOI: 10.1093/biomet/26.4.404.

[40] Clinical and Laboratory Standards Institute. M53-A Criteria for laboratory testing and diagnosis of human immunodeficiency virus infection; approved guideline. Philadelphia (PA): CLSI; 2011.

[41] Le T, Bhushan V, Vasan N. First aid for the USMLE step 1. 20th ed. New York (NY): McGraw-Hill Medical; 2009.

[42] Pereira P, Westgard J, Encarnação P, Seghatchian J. Analytical model for calculating indeterminate results interval of screening tests, the effect on seroconversion window period: A brief evaluation of the impact of uncertain results on the blood establishment budget. Transfus Apher Sci 2014, 51(2):126–131. DOI:10.1016/j.transci.2014.10.004

[43] Fiebig E, Wright D, Rawal B, Garrett P, Schumacher R, et al. Dynamics of HIV viremia and antibody seroconversion in plasma donors: Implications for diagnosis and staging of primary HIV infection. AIDS 2003, 17(13):1871–1879. DOI: 10.1097/00002030-200309050-00005.

[44] Clinical Laboratory Improvement Amendments. CLIA law & regulations. Retrieved from: http://wwwn.cdc.gov/clia/Regulatory/default.aspx. Accessed: March 26, 2016.